A LOVE GREATER THAN DIABETES

A LOVE GREATER THAN DIABETES

AN EMPOWERING GUIDE FOR SUPPORTING CHILDREN WITH TYPE 1 DIABETES

ELIZABETH KILL

Copyright © 2025, Elizabeth Kill

All rights reserved. No part of this book may be used or reproduced by any means, graphic, electronic, or mechanical (including any information storage retrieval system) without the express written permission from the author, except in the case of brief quotations for use in articles and reviews wherein appropriate attribution of the source is made.

Publishing support provided by
Ignite Press
55 Shaw Ave. Suite 204
Clovis, CA 93612
www.IgnitePress.us

ISBN: 979-8-9922009-0-4
ISBN: 979-8-9922009-1-1 (E-book)

For bulk purchases and for booking, contact:

Elizabeth Kill
GreaterthanT1D.com
elizabeth@greaterthan1d.com

Because of the dynamic nature of the Internet, web addresses or links contained in this book may have been changed since publication and may no longer be valid. The content of this book and all expressed opinions are those of the author and do not reflect the publisher or the publishing team. The author is solely responsible for all content included herein.

The author is not a medical professional, and the content in this book is not intended to provide medical advice, diagnosis, or treatment. Consult with your healthcare provider or medical professionals regarding any questions or concerns about managing type 1 diabetes or other medical conditions.

The author and publisher disclaim any liability for any adverse effects resulting from the use of the information contained in this book. This work is meant to inform, inspire, and support, but it should not replace professional medical care or advice.

Library of Congress Control Number: 2024925550

Cover design by Usman Tariq
Edited by Elizabeth Arterberry
Interior design by Jetlaunch

FIRST EDITION

To each of you who walked beside me on this journey, thank you. Your unwavering guidance, support, and encouragement have been the foundation of my strength, fueling my passion to write and emboldening me to share our family's story.

I am deeply grateful for the inspiration you have provided, and it is my hope that this book brings sparks of joy and comfort to the lives of parents and caregivers of newly diagnosed children. May it remind them that they are not alone and that, together, we can hold onto hope, strive for a cure, and look forward to a future of possibility.

TABLE OF CONTENTS

Foreword: Dr. Laurie Marbas ix
Letter to My Reader xi
Chapter 1. 3 a.m.: A Mother's Resilience 1
Chapter 2. Support Squad: Your Circle of Strength 9
Chapter 3. Advocacy in Action: Championing Your Child ... 15
Chapter 4. Embracing Help: Family and Friends in Action... 19
Chapter 5. Heartfelt Help: Grandparents' Journey of Support .. 23
Chapter 6. Sibling Wisdom and Support 29
Chapter 7. Dream Sweetly: Restful Nights with Diabetes 35
Chapter 8. First Getaway: A Breath of Fresh Air 39
Chapter 9. Escape to Napa: A Wild Ride................... 43
Chapter 10. Education Essentials:
  Navigating School with Type 1 Diabetes 47
Chapter 11. Jackson's Diaversary: Celebrating Strength....... 63
Chapter 12. Disney Magic: Managing Type 1 on the Go...... 69
Chapter 13. Super Sitters: Type 1 Tips for Babysitters 73
Chapter 14. Party Prep: Type 1 Birthday Planning Tips 77
Chapter 15. Playdate Pros: Type 1 Tips for Fun 81
Chapter 16. Lakeside Laughter: Our Summer Adventure 85

Chapter 17. Braces, Gummies, and Glucose:
Dental Tips for Type 1 91

Chapter 18. Seasonal Shifts: Insights on Blood Sugar 99

Chapter 19. Diabetes Mastery: The Power of Consistency ... 103

Chapter 20. Happy Holidays: Navigating Festive Times 109

    1. Spooky Fun: Halloween with Type 1 109

    2. Hoppy Days: Easter with Type 1 111

    3. Christmas to Remember 113

Conclusion 117

Appendices 119

    1. Diabetes Decoded: Understanding the Diagnosis 119

    2. Diabetes Dictionary: Your Go-to Glossary 126

    3. Diabetes Unplugged: Back to Basics 129

    4. Tech Talk: Diabetes Devices Explained 131

Resources 135

Acknowledgments 141

About the Author 143

FOREWORD

It's been a true privilege to care for and come to know Elizabeth Kill and her family over the past four years. From our first meeting, Elizabeth's strength, determination, and love for her son, Jackson, who was diagnosed with type 1 diabetes at just four years old, have deeply touched me. Managing a chronic illness like diabetes is no small feat, and Elizabeth has navigated this path with grace, courage, and an unwavering commitment to her child. I've often told her she's the "Mother of the Year" because of the incredible patience, care, and attention she brings to Jackson's daily life.

But what makes Elizabeth truly remarkable is that she's not just focused on her own family. Through her own journey, she's chosen to reach out to others, to share her wisdom and experiences with families who are grappling with a new diagnosis of type 1 diabetes. This book is an extension of the loving, compassionate, and determined person she is. It's filled with the kind of support that only someone who has walked this path can offer—a blend of practical advice, heartfelt encouragement, and the understanding that only another parent in her shoes can give.

Elizabeth didn't just stop at doing everything in her power for Jackson; she made it her mission to help other families facing the same challenges, and that speaks volumes about the person she is. Her book is a gift to those who may feel lost, overwhelmed, or scared. I've watched her grow into a true advocate, and I'm in awe of the way she has turned her family's struggles into a source of hope and strength for others.

It's been an inspiration to witness her journey, and I know this book will be a lifeline for families who need it. I am proud to write this foreword for someone as dedicated, resilient, and selfless as Elizabeth. Her story, her compassion, and her desire to help others are things we can all learn from.

Laurie Marbas, MD, MBA
Board-Certified Family and Lifestyle Medicine Physician

LETTER TO MY READER

If you're holding this book, it's likely because your child was just diagnosed with type 1 diabetes. Right now, you're probably feeling overwhelmed, scared, and maybe a bit lost. I know exactly how you feel because I've been in your shoes. The questions come flooding in: *How do we manage this? What will school look like? How do we handle nights, holidays, or even simple things like playdates? Do we need a CGM or a pump? Will my child really need an injection every time they eat? Will I ever feel comfortable leaving them with a babysitter or going out of town?* It's a whirlwind of worries, and it's hard to know where to even start.

I hear you, and I truly understand. I asked myself those same questions on December 22, 2019, the day my son was diagnosed with type 1 diabetes—a day that will forever be etched in my memory. It's the day our world shifted. The fear was gut-wrenching, the thoughts were nonstop, and the tears flowed uncontrollably. Even now, I can still smell that hospital room, the sterile reminder of the moment our lives took a turn we never anticipated.

In those early days, I threw myself into learning. I read every book I could get my hands on, listened to endless podcasts, and searched high and low for answers to all my burning questions. But something was missing—a mother's voice. I needed someone who had been through this to explain it all in a way that made sense to me as a parent, in the middle of the chaos. That's why I wrote this book. I wanted to create a resource for moms, dads, and caregivers, something that could be your guide as you navigate this new world. A quick reference you can turn to for help, whether you need it for a birthday party, holiday gathering, or just getting through the first few weeks.

I'm here with you through it all. In these pages, you'll find our family's story: the highs, the laughs, and the truly tough moments. I'm sharing them to remind you that you're never alone in this. At the end of the book, there's a resource section with answers to many of the questions I once had. Please remember, this isn't meant to replace medical advice; it simply provides the perspective of a mom who's been where you are right now.

You'll also hear personal insights from my daughter about what it's like having a sibling with type 1 diabetes. I've also included the unwavering support of my parents, who played a vital role in our journey.

The truth is every family's path with type 1 diabetes is different. There's no perfect plan, no one-size-fits-all approach. What matters is that we keep learning from one another and keep pushing forward together. I believe that with hope and determination, we will one day find a cure.

My greatest hope for this book is that it gives you strength; that you'll see that, even in the midst of this challenge, there are moments of joy, growth, and connection for your family.

1
3 A.M.: A MOTHER'S RESILIENCE

It was 3 a.m., and there I was, sitting in a hospital bed, tears streaming down my face. Alarms echoed through the halls, blending with the stark scent of disinfectant—a smell that somehow felt both comforting and oppressive in that moment. I clung to my four-year-old son, Jackson, seeking warmth in the chilling air of the hospital room as he slept peacefully, oblivious to the chaos around us. Nurses bustled in and out, monitoring his blood sugar levels. My mind, operating at half capacity, struggled to absorb the flurry of medical activity. Desperate for answers, I scoured book after book on my phone, naively searching for a cure for his diabetes. I thought I could find a miracle, make an appointment at a renowned place like Cleveland Clinic or Johns Hopkins, and pursue every possible treatment to heal him. But as I delved deeper, trying to understand type 1 diabetes from internet articles, the complexity of it all became overwhelming and utterly exhausting.

Rewind to the week before that chaotic night. I was immersed in the end-of-year rush at work, coordinating with my team to fulfill all our customer orders. Amidst meetings with our accountant to close out the financial year and conducting a physical inventory, I also made sure everyone had scheduled time off for the Christmas holiday.

My husband was equally swamped, managing his businesses while planning our holiday events and wrapping up gifts. We were juggling everything perfectly, looking forward to a fantastic Christmas and a surprise post-holiday trip to an indoor waterpark with the kids.

However, throughout that week, Jackson began showing unusual signs. He wet the bed every night and was unusually lethargic. Assuming it was a virus making him too tired to wake up, I waited a few days. By Sunday morning, my concern outweighed my optimism. I decided to call the pediatrician, not wanting to risk spreading any illness at the upcoming family gatherings. After hearing about Jackson's symptoms, the pediatrician urged us to visit urgent care for a blood sugar test through a urine sample.

Unsure of the reason but trusting the advice, I threw on a baseball cap and sweatshirt and drove Jackson to a nearby children's urgent care. They quickly ushered us into a room. As a germaphobe, I found myself sanitizing our hands religiously while we waited for the doctor. He listened to the symptoms and my recount of the pediatrician's advice, then asked for a urine sample.

Getting Jackson to cooperate in the public restroom of the hospital—used by countless sick visitors—was a struggle. I tried explaining that it was just like peeing outside or in the toilet, but he was adamant. "No, I don't want to pee in a cup," he protested.

Despite my frustration and attempts at bribery, it took 45 minutes. I can't even recall what finally convinced him, but he did it. I handed the sample to the nurse and waited in the room, sanitizing every surface once more, driven by a mix of relief and anxiety.

The doctor reappeared, his tone grave. "His blood sugar was 542. We need to transfer him immediately to the main campus of Nationwide Children's Hospital. You can either take him straight there or we can send you in a squad. He might need to stay there for about three days."

My mind reeled as he spoke, the numbers and words swirling into an indecipherable fog. Over 500? What did that mean? I pride myself on being well-informed, yet I stood there, baffled and frightened. Why did we need to rush to another hospital? Couldn't they just treat him here and let us go home?

The room felt colder as the doctor left, but then the nurse came in, her presence warm and comforting. Trying to hold back tears, I asked her to explain everything again. Her gentle voice was like a steady hand on my shoulder. "Elizabeth, please go grab Jackson's favorite stuffed animal, his pillow, a blanket, and some clothes, and head straight to the children's hospital."

The floodgates opened as she spoke. Despite my efforts to stay composed for Jackson's sake, tears streamed down my face. He sat quietly, watching me with wide, uncertain eyes. I picked him up, feeling his small arms wrap around me, his head resting on my shoulder—a silent exchange of love and comfort as we walked to the car.

Strapping him into his seat, I dialed my husband, but my words were muffled by sobs. After a few deep breaths, I managed to explain the situation. "We are headed home, can you pack Jackson's things? Please call my mom to pick up Marlee Kate; we need to head to Children's now and may be there for a few days."

I pulled into our driveway—which is a moment that is engraved in my mind—I turned off the engine, and ran straight into my husband's waiting arms, hoping that I would suddenly wake up from this dream. Marlee Kate, our daughter, stood teary-eyed on the steps of the garage, confused and scared by the sight of her mom and dad enveloped in such raw sorrow. It was a piercing reminder of how quickly life can pivot, thrusting us into realms of fear and uncertainty we never expected to navigate.

My husband, Todd, hastily loaded the car, while my mom arrived to pick up our anxious Marlee Kate, who, despite her confusion, found solace in knowing she'd be with Nana and Papa. We then sped towards the children's hospital, perhaps a little too fast, as urgency gripped our every action.

Upon arriving, Jackson found brief joy playing on a gigantic turtle sculpture in the lobby—a welcome distraction that brought a smile to his face. At that moment, my usual vigilance over germs slipped away; my mind was consumed with trying to understand the implications of what the urgent care doctor had said.

The staff at Nationwide Children's Hospital were nothing short of incredible. They expedited our check-in process, ushering us to our room swiftly, which we reached by 3 p.m. It was there, in that small, sterile room, that I finally allowed myself to take a deep breath. Todd, ever attentive, reminded me to grab something to eat. "It's going to be a long night, and you need to keep your strength up," he said gently.

Eating was the last thing on my mind, but he was right—I needed to be strong, not just for Jackson, but for myself, too. In that whirlwind of emotions, it felt nearly impossible to take care of myself without fearing that I might miss an important update or decision about Jackson's care. The weight of everything hung heavily.

At exactly 4:12 p.m., the medical team sprang into action. They entered swiftly, immediately setting up to draw blood for various tests, administer insulin, and initiate educational briefings. My mind was awash with questions, my manufacturing background driving my need to understand every detail. What is the underlying cause of this disease? How can it be cured? What factors increase or decrease blood sugar? Why is there such variability in the condition? What is the safe range we need to maintain? I had countless more questions, but the doctor provided only a brief overview, reassuring me that everything would be alright and that I would learn more during our stay. Despite the reassurance, I was eager to absorb all the information I could to expedite our departure.

As Jackson contentedly ate two popsicles given to him by the nurse, he nestled against his favorite stuffed kitty cat and a blue-starred pillow on the hospital bed. Meanwhile, my husband and I pored over the information provided, delving into further research. The vastness of the internet offered an overwhelming amount of information, making it challenging to discern what was relevant to our situation. The digital maze was intriguing but dangerous, threatening to pull us down countless rabbit holes if we weren't careful.

About an hour later, a man arrived with a cart filled with wooden toys and pots of paint, igniting a spark of joy in Jackson's eyes. He warmly encouraged Jackson to choose any toy and paint it in any colors he liked. Turning to me with wide eyes, Jackson asked, "Can I really paint this wooden truck right here in bed?"

"Yes, Jackson, you can," I assured him.

His face lit up with sheer joy, a welcome distraction, especially when another nurse came in to draw his blood again to check his glucose levels, which were thankfully decreasing to the 300s. When the nurse offered me the chance to do the finger poke, my initial hesitation gave way to determination. Unsure but ready, I thought, *No better time than the present. Let's do this.*

I became a diligent scribe, jotting down everything and bombarding the nurses with endless questions every time they checked on Jackson. My focus was sharp on his numbers—understanding what they were and where they needed to be was crucial for when we would eventually go home. In an attempt to make sense of it all, I started charting everything in Excel. It might seem excessive, but I was desperate to detect any patterns or themes that could explain the fluctuations in his condition. At that time, I didn't realize that understanding his baseline and correction factor was essential before making any further assumptions. All I knew that I could do then was research and document diligently. That was my way of coping with the situation as it happened.

After the final check of the night, my husband returned home to get some sleep while I stayed behind, snuggling with Jackson as we watched TV until he drifted off to sleep. Despite my exhaustion, my adrenaline kept me wide awake, my mind racing with concerns about managing our day-to-day life. How would we handle daycare? What about my business? The sheer volume of changes we needed to navigate felt overwhelming, too immense to fully grasp at that moment.

For the next two days, our lives revolved around a rigorous schedule of checks every two hours, each session punctuated by lessons on managing insulin dosages and calculating carbohydrates. Amidst the clinical routine, Jackson found solace and a bit of normalcy in darting off to choose a new toy from the hospital's toy room during breaks. His favorite was the Hot Wheels track set up by the window in our room, where he could momentarily forget the hospital setting. We also learned to handle the terrifying emergencies of sudden glucose drops or spikes during the quiet of the night.

Desperate for some semblance of control, I pushed for a continuous glucose monitor, hoping it would bring us precision and peace of mind. However, the response was a firm "no;" we were told we must first master the manual basics for six months. The prospect of enduring half a year without technological assistance was overwhelming. Sleep became a distant memory, replaced by constant anxiety. How could I ensure his safety every moment? How could I possibly manage this new reality?

My husband held my hand, looked into my eyes, and reassured me, "We can do this, together. It won't be easy, but we're strong and we'll learn and adjust as we go."

His words brought me comfort as we faced the unknown. Then, on the morning of Christmas Eve, which marked the third day at Children's, our doctor brought us news: we could go home that afternoon. My heart leapt with joy—I couldn't wait to return home, to hold my sweet Marlee Kate, whom I missed terribly, and to be in our own space for Christmas. As we were leaving, I noticed hospital staff bringing Christmas trees into each room on the endocrinology floor. A pang of guilt washed over me; while we were going home, other families would still be here over the holidays. This sight deeply moved me, and by our fourth year navigating our new reality, a spark of joy came over us and we found our own way to give back to those spending their Christmas on the endocrinology floor.

> My husband held my hand, looked into my eyes, and reassured me, "We can do this, together. It won't be easy, but we're strong and we'll learn and adjust as we go."

♡ Advice:

I want to reassure you from the heart—everything will eventually be okay. There truly is light at the end of this tunnel. Embarking on this journey is daunting; there's so much to learn. It's crucial to begin with the basics. Understanding the foundational elements allows you to build a robust knowledge base. Although technology offers great help, it isn't infallible. Even when I was determined to convince the doctor to let us use a continuous glucose monitor (CGM) sooner, I realized she was right. I needed to grasp the essentials first.

That said, it's worth mentioning that I didn't follow the recommended six-month wait; I only waited two. What matters the most is learning how to calculate carbs and figure out your correction factor, which can make each day and every meal more manageable. Some days will flow smoothly, while others may be unexpectedly challenging. It's tough, but finding a community that understands and supports you is crucial. I'll share specific tools and resources in this book, but connecting with those who have experienced this journey firsthand will undoubtedly make your path lighter.

2

SUPPORT SQUAD: YOUR CIRCLE OF STRENGTH

Have you ever felt alone, isolated, lost, and unsure of what the days ahead would look like? I felt all of that after we left the hospital. It was as if, in just two days, my world had turned upside down. I lost control of everything, not knowing what to do next. This overwhelming feeling hit me hard and fast. I knew I couldn't sort it out on my own quickly. I needed a community. I needed support, guidance, and reassurance that everything would be okay. But reaching out for help was one of the hardest things for me as an introvert.

> I will never forget her first message to me. She let me know everything was going to be okay and that she was available to help in any way she could. Little did she know I would have a million-plus questions for her.

My journey began with an introduction from another mom who had two children with type 1 diabetes. I will never forget her first message to me. She let me know everything was going to be okay and that she was available to help in any way she could. Little did she know I would have a million-plus questions for her. Within an hour of her initial text, I was messaging her about everything: how much insulin to give for different meals; what it means when blood sugar goes high after two hours; how many carbs to give when my child is low; favorite low snacks; calculating carbs in processed foods; understanding what a correction ratio was, and so much more.

The questions kept coming for months, but gradually, they became less frequent. During that initial period, I felt incredibly blessed to have her time and guidance. It was truly a spark of joy! My husband also jumped into the fray, researching Facebook communities centered around type 1 diabetes, gathering information on the best scales for counting carbs, checking blood sugar at night without waking our child, and understanding meal intervals. While the online community was very supportive and helped us navigate these rocky waters, the sheer volume of information was overwhelming. It's essential to be cautious and not get lost in endless research.

♡ Advice:

Building the right community is an evolving process, depending on where you are in your journey. Just like any community, there are many types of personalities—some strong, some shy, some funny, and some always positive. When you start developing your community, it's essential to find your kind of people. Who do you relate to the most? This will guide you in connecting with those who align with your values and approach to life. This applies to choosing an endocrinologist, a nutritionist, a teacher at school, your Facebook groups, or the people you follow on Instagram. You want your community to resonate with you and how you view the world. For me, I prefer to look at life with a positive outlook, knowing that there is always something to learn or gain from each interaction. There is no perfect size or number. The only important thing is that someone is there for you: in hard times, to lift you up, and in good times, to celebrate with you!

Today, I now have an amazing physician, a moms group, and a great friend who I can reach out to at any time to get advice or vent, and I surround myself with positive people who are aligned with finding a cure.

Tips:

From my perspective, there are a few key communities that are essential:

Another Caregiver:
- Finding another caregiver you can connect with and text at any time is invaluable. This person may be introduced to you by a friend or someone you meet at a type 1 function or event. I still text my friend about new challenges and changes, seeking her advice. She provides comfort and understanding when nights are hard and supports me as we continually research and explore ways to support our children.

A Good Endocrinologist:
- Sometimes, you may not have a choice, depending on your insurance, but if you do, make sure your goals align with theirs. You don't want to be in a situation where your doctor isn't focusing on what's important for you and your child.

Online Community:
- While the online community can be incredibly supportive, jumping into Facebook can reveal numerous communities and information that could take days, weeks, or even months to sift through. Later in this chapter, I list a few

groups that I like to follow because the information they share is relevant, and they strive to keep things positive and uplifting.

Events and Organizations:
- Organizations like Friends for Life, Breakthrough T1, Beyond Type 1, and Mastering Diabetes host events either online or locally in the community. These events provide amazing opportunities to meet other parents and for your child to meet other kids their age who also are living with type 1. These events include educational sessions, social activities, and opportunities to build lasting friendships with others who understand the challenges of living with type 1 diabetes.

Organizations:

Breakthrough T1D (formerly JDRF): They have local chapters across the U.S. that provide support and resources for people with type 1 diabetes. You can connect with your local chapter through their website (Breakthrough T1D).

Beyond Type 1: This organization offers a variety of support options, including online communities and resources for people with type 1 diabetes. They also provide mental health resources specifically tailored to the needs of the type 1 diabetes community (Beyond Type 1).

Children with Diabetes (CWD): "Friends for Life" conferences and events provide a space where children, teens, adults, and families affected by type 1 diabetes can connect, share experiences, and find support and education tailored to their needs. These events include educational sessions, social activities, and opportunities to build lasting friendships with others who understand the challenges of living with type 1 diabetes.

American Diabetes Association (ADA): ADA has a support directory and local offices that can help connect you with peer support groups in your area.

Facebook Groups

- Juicebox Podcast: Type 1 Diabetes
- Elementary and Diabetes
- Mastering Diabetes Kids Club
- Poked – Parents of Kids Enduring Diabetes

These are just a few of the many organizations and communities you can join. I will have more listed in my resource page if you're interested.

3

ADVOCACY IN ACTION: CHAMPIONING YOUR CHILD

After 72 hours of training and education at Nationwide Children's, my husband and I were completely exhausted and overwhelmed with information. We learned how to inject insulin, where to inject it, how many hours to wait before the next meal, and so much more. Yet, after a few days at home, countless new questions kept arising. We eagerly awaited our upcoming endocrinology appointment, hoping for more insights and support. I meticulously documented every event since Jackson was admitted to the hospital, determined to educate myself as thoroughly as possible.

Unfortunately, the visit was disappointing. Besides learning about the importance of occasional indulgences like pizza and cupcakes, we walked away without any deeper understanding of how to manage Jackson's condition effectively. It became clear that while this endocrinologist might be a good fit for some, she wasn't the right fit for us.

As parents, advocating for our children is one of our most vital roles. Initially, I relied heavily on the expertise of professionals, trusting they knew best. However, I quickly learned that understanding and navigating various perspectives and Jackson's unique needs is crucial. I wanted to make sure that we found a medical professional that could dive in deeper and who was aligned with our goals for Jackson.

In the school system, advocating for Jackson has been essential as well. Fortunately, we have a supportive team of teachers and an amazing leader who are committed to helping Jackson thrive. However, I know not everyone has this experience.

> Type 1 diabetes is not a "one-size-fits-all" condition. You might prefer one insulin or glucose monitor over another, or none at all, and that's okay. Trust yourself and your child. You're the best advocate they have.

When Jackson started school, we requested a meeting with the principal, guidance counselor, and nurse to discuss how we manage his type 1 diabetes. We provided a detailed overview of his condition, lifestyle changes, personality, and our management approach. We also asked for a teacher who would be a good fit for Jackson's personality. For example, a shy child might not do well with a teacher who is very vocal about his diabetes, as it could make him more introverted. All these little things can make such a difference in your child's experience. I know there are some parents I have spoken with that had a difficult experience and decided to homeschool their child. There isn't a one-size-fits-all approach. Each situation is unique.

Remember, you know what is best for your child. Don't rush into any big decisions until you and your child are ready. I'm often asked why Jackson isn't on a pump yet, but it's just not the right fit for us right now, and it may never be. Type 1 diabetes is not a "one-size-fits-all" condition. You might prefer one insulin or glucose monitor over another, or none at all, and that's okay. Trust yourself and your child. You're the best advocate they have.

Key Points for Advocacy

- Preparation and Documentation: Arrive at medical appointments with detailed documentation to track patterns and facilitate informed discussions with healthcare providers.
- Finding the Right Fit: Not all professionals will align with your approach. Seek a second opinion or find a provider who better understands your needs.
- Comprehensive Care: Advocate for discussions on holistic management strategies, including lifestyle changes and mental health support.
- Proactive Communication: Set up meetings with school staff at the beginning of the school year to discuss your child's needs and ensure they are paired with a supportive teacher.
- Building Relationships: Establish a good relationship with the school team for better cooperation and support.
- Trusting Your Instincts: Make decisions based on what feels right for your child, rather than external pressures.

Your experience underscores the importance of being an informed, proactive, and assertive advocate for your child in all areas of life. Each child's needs and circumstances are different, and personalized care and support are crucial in managing type 1 diabetes effectively.

♡ Advice:

My advice is to always trust your intuition and always ask questions. There is never a dumb question that is asked. My father always says, "the more you learn, the more opportunities you have in life." This is so true, especially with regard to educating yourself to make the best decisions for your child.

Tips:

When meeting with any professional, make sure you have an outline of what you would like to discuss. Examples include:

- What do I do when I start seeing highs at night?
- What are the benefits of a CGM and/or pump?
- What markers should I be keeping an eye on for my child?
- Where are the best places to inject insulin?
- What types of insulins are available and what would be best for my child?
- Do you provide education for grandparents or caregivers in your office?
- How do I get a hold of someone if my child becomes ill? Who will walk me through the steps? What things do I need to look out for?
- What forms do I need to have for school or daycare?

If you are in a tough situation and not sure where to go next, you can always send a question out to your community for advice. I would not use any personal names or the business' name to ensure privacy.

4

EMBRACING HELP: FAMILY AND FRIENDS IN ACTION

Are you someone who's always juggling multiple tasks, thinking that if you just stay up for one more hour, you can get everything done? But then it never seems to happen, and your sleep suffers as a result. As much as you might want to be superwoman, it's just not feasible.

I've never been one to ask for much help. I've always been the type to juggle my schedule, making sure the kids are where they need to be and staying up late to handle things around the house. But this approach often results in me neglecting my own needs. However, when our world was turned upside down, my perspective shifted completely, and the joy that came from this new lens was truly incredible.

The moment we learned we were headed to Nationwide Children's Hospital, my husband sprang into action. He reached out to our family and friends, asking for their prayers and support for our son, Jackson. The response we received was beyond anything I could have imagined.

The first message came from a friend whose child attended daycare with Jackson. She offered to spend time with Jackson while my husband and I were in class, learning about our son's condition.

The second message was from a neighbor, offering to wrap all our Christmas gifts so we wouldn't have to worry about it when we were released from the hospital on Christmas Eve. It was an incredibly thoughtful gesture that touched our hearts.

The third message came from my family, updating us on our daughter, who was with them, and offering to bring us dinner from our favorite restaurants.

The fourth message was from my husband's family, offering to come and stay with us to help out while we adjusted to our new reality.

The fifth message was from my colleagues at work, assuring me that they had everything covered and encouraging me to focus on my family during this challenging time.

The sixth message was from one of my college roommates, offering valuable advice based on her own experience with medical issues.

> We came home to a huge poster that one of the neighbors purchased and took around to all our neighbors so they could write messages to Jackson about how they loved him and to tell him that he was such a warrior.

Many more messages of encouragement and prayers poured in, bringing tears to my eyes each time I read them. Even now, as I write this at my local coffee shop, I find myself overcome with emotion.

Lastly, when we arrived home from the hospital on December 24, we came home to a huge poster that one of the neighbors purchased and took around to all our neighbors so they could write messages to Jackson about how they loved him and to tell him that he was such a warrior. It brought so much joy to him and our whole family to feel such love.

♡ Advice:

If you ever find yourself wanting to help someone in need, remember that heartfelt words carry more meaning than you might realize. And when it's your turn to receive help, as difficult as it may be, embrace it. Say "yes" to those who are eager and willing to support you.

Tips:

- For a kiddo, being in the hospital can be lonely, so offer to bring them their favorite pillow, stuffed animal, and a change of clothes.
- If there are siblings, offer to help care for them and support them during the duration of their sibling's stay in the hospital.
- Emotional support and texts are great, but getting a phone call and hearing someone's voice, and being able to talk through all the emotions, means so much.
- Food, if you are one that likes to make dinners and drop them off, is always great. Just check in with the family about what they may like, as adjusting to new foods and ratios can be challenging.
- Remember, asking for help is a sign of strength, not weakness. It takes courage to reach out, and accepting support from others can make all the difference in overcoming challenges. Don't hesitate to seek or receive help when you need it.

5

HEARTFELT HELP: GRANDPARENTS' JOURNEY OF SUPPORT

Introduction:

When life throws us unexpected challenges, the ripple effects extend far beyond our own experience. Our struggles, joys, and every moment in between are shared with the people we love, whether they are family by blood or the close friends we consider family. In times of joy, they celebrate with us, and in times of hardship, they carry our burdens. That's why I felt it was important to share my parents' journey with you, so you can see the world through the eyes of caregivers who often take on more than we realize in our most difficult moments.

In this chapter, my parents talk about how they managed during this time, and how, despite the challenges, they discovered their own sparks of joy. My father, in particular, found a new passion he never knew he had in cooking. He's now using this passion to create special memories with the kids, turning mealtimes into moments of comfort and connection. Because, in the end, there's nothing more heartwarming than breaking bread with the ones you love.

My mother, lovingly known as Nurse Nana, stepped into the role of caregiver with grace and devotion. She supported Jackson through his injections, offering encouragement and reassurance at every turn, always finding ways to bring joy into the most difficult moments. Whether through her loving care or her warm smile, she made sure Jackson felt both comforted and uplifted during a time when he needed it most.

A Letter from the Grandparents

Have you ever received a phone call in which your child is crying so hard that you can't even recognize their voice? That's the call my husband and I got on December 22. It was the day we found out our grandchild had been diagnosed with type 1 diabetes.

In that moment, a whirlwind of thoughts raced through our minds. Is this permanent? What is this disease? How will it affect Jackson? Why did this happen to our grandchild? How can we fix it, and what can we do to help?

We immediately reached out to family members and friends who had children with type 1 diabetes and started researching how we could support him. We attended a class at the endocrinologist's office to grasp what this diagnosis truly meant. Our understanding shifted from a broad overview to an in-depth, daily learning experience.

When Jackson came home, the reality set in. He was only four years old, and every time we had to help with finger pricks, he would scream and cry, begging us not to do it. As grandparents, this was heart-wrenching and far from anything we ever imagined we'd have to do. At the same time, our daughter was running herself ragged managing her business, taking care of Jackson, and supporting her family. We were deeply concerned about her well-being, the family's stability, and their marriage.

This experience was a turning point for us. We realized our role as grandparents had profoundly changed. It wasn't just about changing diapers and handing out lollipops anymore. It was about stepping up to something greater—being a pillar of support in a challenging and unexpected journey. Here are five ways we stepped up that may be helpful to you and your family.

One way my husband stepped up was by cooking for Jackson and the family. He poured himself into researching which plants would be most beneficial for stabilizing blood sugar, down to the specifics of certain roots, like konjac root. Our daughter decided to switch the entire family to a plant-based lifestyle, and my husband embraced this challenge wholeheartedly.

> It was about stepping up to something greater—being a pillar of support in a challenging and unexpected journey.

He began experimenting with soups: some turned out fantastic, while others were so bad they went straight to the garbage disposal. But he didn't give up. He kept trying, creating a variety of soups, burritos, and wraps. Some of these dishes really helped in stabilizing Jackson's blood sugar. We discovered that beans are truly remarkable. It also changed the way my husband eats and fuels his body as a result.

For those who know my husband, this transformation was extraordinary. Cooking had never been his thing. If you're reading this and thinking, *I don't know how to cook*, just remember that my husband was in the same boat. He had never cooked before. It was a completely new experience for him, but he dove in headfirst, determined to support our family in any way he could. His dedication and love shone through every meal he made, helping us navigate this unexpected journey together.

Another way we supported Jackson was by learning how to manage his diabetes. We educated ourselves on checking blood sugar levels and administering insulin. This included both Humalog, which is fast-acting, and Lantus, which is long-acting. It took us four years to reach the final step of being able to change out his Dexcom, the continuous glucose monitor.

By mastering these skills, we could provide hands-on support. Learning to check his blood sugar and give injections was daunting at first, but it became second nature over time. It allowed us to share the burden with our daughter and ensure Jackson always had the care he needed. This commitment to learning and adapting was another crucial way we supported our family during this challenging time.

We also made sure that our home was a place that Jackson wanted to be. So, whenever he came over, we dropped everything and spent time doing kid stuff and learning along the way. This was a great joy to both my husband and me. Having our home feel like a comfort zone for him allowed his parents to drop him off anytime, to carry on with their lives, and to support their daughter so she could feel normal and not worry about her brother as much.

Learning to balance food intake to manage his blood sugar levels was another task that took some trial and error. One thing we learned by adjusting food when he was low, was to wait long enough for the food to have an impact—about 5 to 10 minutes—before taking any additional action to bring up his numbers. On the high side, we learned that drinking water and doing exercises was a way to bring down his numbers slowly, but without insulin. So, we did a lot of jumping jacks together or had a contest involving the number of times we could run around the house. This helped us realize just how out of shape we were.

Today, we read anything that comes across our desk about type 1 diabetes. Our biggest point of interest is in the future development of ways to reactivate the pancreas so that, just maybe, someday Jackson can live his life without insulin. The blessing of his disease has been him learning about and enjoying a plant-based nutritional lifestyle, which has been the result of a loving family. We're sure he will carry on his plant-based lifestyle in ways that will make us very proud of his journey to living his best life.

♡ Advice:

In conclusion, every grandparent finds their unique way to help their children and grandchildren navigate challenging times. My dad, a former executive who had never cooked a day in his life, rolled up his sleeves and jumped right in, finding his spark of joy in cooking for us. He drops off meals when life gets hectic. My mom, always with a warm smile, is ready to help in any way she can, even when she's unsure. I feel truly blessed to have such amazing parents to support and lean on. Their love and dedication are the foundation that helps us all through this journey.

Tips:

Ways to support your child and their spouse in the beginning:

- Offer to babysit; maybe start with a couple hours, and move up to an overnight!
- Offer to go to the grocery or run other errands.
- Help out one night with monitoring blood sugar.

6
SIBLING WISDOM AND SUPPORT

When Jackson was diagnosed with type 1 diabetes, I didn't immediately grasp how much it would ripple through our entire family, especially affecting his sister, Marlee Kate. She has always been incredibly empathetic and caring, but it took time for me to realize just how deeply this journey had impacted her. Wanting to give voice to the often-overlooked emotional journey that siblings go through, I asked Marlee Kate to share her own thoughts and experiences.

In my resource guide, I've included a list of questions you can use to spark conversations with your other children. It's so important to open the dialogue now, as they may have emotions or concerns they're not comfortable expressing on their own. By bringing these questions up, you create a space for them to share things they may not have felt ready to ask, helping to strengthen your family's emotional resilience while continuing on this journey.

I have summarized her thoughts and feelings to give you an idea of what you may want to think about with your own sibling children and the questions you may want to ask them.

1. **Marlee Kate's Initial Reaction**

   How did you feel when you first heard about your brother's diagnosis?

   I was scared because I didn't know what was happening to my brother.

   What was your immediate concern or question?

   My biggest worry was why my brother was going to the hospital and whether he was going to be okay. I was only in first grade, and I was so concerned that I felt sick every day from worrying.

2. **Understanding Diabetes**

   How did you learn about type 1 diabetes and what it means for your brother?

   I watched documentaries on type 1 to understand it better. Over time, I slowly started to grasp what it meant for Jackson.

   Was there anything that surprised you about the condition?

   I was really surprised that he got it. After a sleepover, I remember feeling tired and thinking Jackson had caught something like the flu. When my mom said we needed to take Jackson to the doctor, I didn't think it was serious until they had to go to Children's Hospital. I helped pack his things, but I didn't fully understand what was happening until later.

3. **Family Dynamics**

   How do you think your brother's diagnosis has affected our family as a whole?

   It's changed a lot about how and what we eat, which I think is good for our health. Before, I used to get sick often, but now, we hardly ever get sick. I believe our diet has made our immune systems stronger.

   Have there been any changes in your relationship with him?

   I definitely care for him more now. I check in on him often, especially when we argue—I'll check his numbers because if he's low, he might be sad, and if he's high, he might be mad or irritable. Even though I know our parents are here to take care of him, I still worry, but not as much as I used to.

4. **Daily Life**

   How has your brother's daily routine changed since his diagnosis?

   He can't eat as much as before and he's more private about his condition. He doesn't want people to know or talk about it, like when his cousins were over, and he didn't want to explain what "bolus" meant. I just said it was one of his stuffed animals to end the conversation.

   Are there any new responsibilities you've taken on?

   I keep an eye on his numbers and make sure he's not eating anything that could harm him. At school, I depend on the nurse to help, but I always want to be there if he needs anything.

5. **Emotional Impact**

   How has his diagnosis affected you emotionally?

   It's made me more aware of how things can change and I still worry a lot because I don't want anything bad to happen to him.

   Have you found any ways to cope, or to support him?

   Being closer to him helps me understand his situation better. If he's okay, then I'm okay.

6. **Role and Support**

   In what ways have you tried to support your brother?

   I help manage his numbers with food, which is really important.

   How do you feel your role in the family has changed, if at all?

   I'll always be the big sister, but now I'm more protective and aware of what he needs.

7. **Challenges and Triumphs**

   What challenges have you noticed your brother facing?

   He can't eat whatever he wants or do everything he used to. Sleepovers are tough because he can't manage his numbers at night, so it's easier to have them at our house where we can help.

   Can you share any proud moments or achievements since his diagnosis?

   In the beginning, he couldn't leave the house much, but now he's more independent. Recently, he even started giving himself his own insulin.

8. **Learning and Growth**

   What have you learned about resilience and strength from your brother's experience?

   I've learned that you should never give up, even when times are hard.

   How has this experience changed your perspective on health and family?

   I've learned that you are what you eat. Eating well makes you feel better, and this experience has made me realize how much our family cares for each other. We all do our best to help out.

9. **Hopes and Wishes**

   What are your hopes for your brother's future?

   I hope he continues to take care of himself.

   What advice would you give to other siblings in similar situations?

   When times are tough, don't give up. Your parents might not get much sleep, so help out as much as you can. It gets better over time.

10. Final Thoughts

Is there anything else you'd like to share about this journey?

I think our whole family is more aware of good eating habits and how they affect our health.

How do you think this experience will shape our family moving forward?

It will make us a better family by learning more about diseases, health, food, and exercise. I'm really proud of my parents for being there for my brother during such tough times.

7

DREAM SWEETLY: RESTFUL NIGHTS WITH DIABETES

Sleep. This five-letter word is one of the pillars of longevity and a healthy life. It is tied to our performance, productivity, development, immune function, hormonal balance, and so much more. As many of you are reading this, you're probably thinking, *Great, but how am I going to get my sleep?*

I understand your concern all too well. The night Jackson was diagnosed, I sat in the hospital with a million thoughts racing through my mind. *Am I going to be waking up every two hours for the rest of my life? Will I ever be able to sleep for eight hours without an alarm or without worrying about his blood sugar levels?*

•••••••••••••••••••

Am I going to be waking up every two hours for the rest of my life? Will I ever be able to sleep for eight hours without an alarm or without worrying about his blood sugar levels?

•••••••••••••••••••

Many nights we would wake up at 2:30 a.m., put our headlamp on, five test strips laid out, hands washed, moving Jackson ever so slightly so he didn't wake up. Finally, we got a finger stick, but the meter timed out. So, we reset. By the time we reset, the blood dried. Start over. Then, the test strips fell on the floor because we bumped them. This was my husband and me for the first three months. It was comical at times, and just exhausting on some nights. But, wow, you learn so much each night, and you start to develop a system to streamline it and make it faster.

Each person has their own way of monitoring their child's blood sugar through the night. Some continue with finger pokes, others use a Continuous Glucose Monitor (CGM), and some have a CGM and pump. Each method offers different benefits and can ease the day or the evening for the child with type 1 diabetes, depending on how you manage it. I can speak very closely about using a CGM, as we switched after several months of finger pokes. If you are new to this, it's good to weigh the benefits of each. It takes time with any method to get into a rhythm. If you want more information, you can see my resource page for more details.

Despite the challenges, these experiences taught us resilience and the importance of sleep. Every night, we got better at it. Each routine became more efficient, and we discovered small adjustments that made a big difference. Now, looking back, I realize how crucial those sleep-deprived nights were in shaping our journey.

There are many variables that come into play when your kiddo goes to bed—from what they ate to hormones, growth spurts, exercise, and sickness. You can only manage so much, and some nights are better than others. Just take it one night at a time.

Regardless of which method you choose, it's crucial to find support. Having a partner or a reliable person who can give you a night off to watch your kiddo's blood sugar is so important.

♡ Advice:

These experiences taught us resilience and the importance of a good night's sleep. Each night, we became more efficient, discovering small adjustments that made a big difference. Looking back, I realize how crucial those sleep-deprived nights were in shaping our journey. Remember, you're not alone. Take it one night at a time, find a system that works for you, and seek support when needed. Together, we can navigate these nighttime challenges and ensure better sleep for both you and your child.

Tips:

- Finding a system that works for you and your family is important. Is there someone who can help monitor your child's blood glucose level one day a week in the evening?
- If I can, I try to have a very clean dinner that is very predictable and won't create a high later in the evening. If you are looking for ideas on clean dinners, I have provided a few of our favorites in the resource section.
- If possible, we try to eat at least two hours before bed. That way, I know where his blood sugar level will be heading into the evening.
- Sugar Pixel has a great device that is easy to use that will alert you and monitor your kiddo's blood sugar numbers (our school even got one to keep a close eye on Jackson's numbers).
- A bedtime routine is a perfect opportunity to carve out even just 5 minutes to listen to something calming, read a book, or practice deep breathing before sleep.
- Exercise after dinner is amazing, not just for your kiddo living with type 1 diabetes, but also for the whole family. It is shown that exercise (walking, jogging, jumping on the trampoline, etc) can help your body use insulin more effectively for all

people living with type 1 diabetes or not. One of the kids' favorite things to do after dinner is go on a bike ride, which can be a nice win; as I clean up dinner in peace, they are off exercising!

8

FIRST GETAWAY: A BREATH OF FRESH AIR

Are you feeling completely exhausted? Did you manage to get enough sleep last night? Can you count the hours of sleep you got not just on one hand, but on both? Perhaps during your university years, or in those early days with a newborn, you might have thought those sleep-deprived nights were firmly in the past.

Yet, here I was, far from the clear, as the doctor outlined the risks and potential repercussions if Jackson's blood sugar was not meticulously managed. Those initial weeks were filled with fear and anxiety; sleep evaded me as I grappled with uncertainty. The pressing question that haunted my nights: was this the new normal?

> I felt like I was an on-call nurse with no end to my shift.

Fast forward a year, and while things were improving, the challenges persisted. I felt like I was an on-call nurse with no end to my shift. I took on this perpetual vigilance by choice, driven by the belief that no one else could care for him quite like I could. And the thought of letting go, of trusting others, seeded a fear that it might only add to my sleeplessness. I couldn't have been more mistaken.

I regret not embracing the offers from family and friends who were willing to lend a hand, to let me catch up on sleep without the constant need to monitor glucose levels, to give me a night off from the cycle of checking, correcting, and feeding. But, eventually, I hit a wall.

It was then that my parents intervened, insisting I needed to step away, if only for a night, to rest and rejuvenate. Despite my hesitations, I recognized the necessity of being my best self for Jackson, and so, with a heart heavy with trepidation, I departed for a weekend rendezvous with college friends—a six-hour drive from home. Was this a leap too far?

The initial evening was peppered with check-ins, but I gradually settled into the flow, confident in the plans I'd laid out for his care. For the first time in what seemed like an eternity, I fully immersed myself in the joy of companionship. We reminisced, laughed heartily, and caught up on each other's lives, allowing the warmth of friendship to surround me.

By the weekend's end, the rejuvenation I felt was profound. My parents had excelled in their role, managing everything. This experience bolstered my confidence, and I returned home with a renewed spirit, knowing that Jackson was in capable hands and that help was just a call away.

♡ Advice:

Every caregiver, regardless of who they care for, needs to embrace the necessity of stepping back occasionally. It doesn't require an elaborate getaway; sometimes, just a couple of hours spent wandering the aisles of Target or sinking into the uninterrupted peace of a nap can work wonders. Your body and mind both require this time to rejuvenate. When we allow ourselves these pauses, the benefits are many. There's a restoration of energy, a decluttering of the mind, and a revitalization of the spirit. It's remarkable how a short span of solitude can impart such a profound sense of renewal.

Tips:

- Establishing a support system is critical. Perhaps there's a trusted friend, a family member, a neighbor, or even a community volunteer who can step in to provide that necessary break. Aim for a regular interval—monthly or even quarterly—to ensure you're giving yourself this essential care.
- Reach out to other moms in the diabetes community you are in to see if they know of any babysitters that are trained to help support you.

9

ESCAPE TO NAPA: A WILD RIDE

You're either a travel enthusiast, exploring the world at every opportunity, or you prefer to stay close to home, surrounded by friends and family. Since graduating college, I've embraced every chance to wander. Whether it's a trip with loved ones or adventures with friends, I've been there. As my career began to flourish, I eagerly jumped on planes to visit customers or suppliers. Then we had kids, and while it slowed down a bit, the urge to explore was always there. So, when I turned 40, my husband surprised me with a trip to Napa, California, with a few friends. I was over the moon, excited to go, but also nervous about leaving Jackson for the first time.

As we approached the trip, my planning went into overdrive. I created a binder for my parents. Yes, a binder. It outlined each day with the kids' activities and meal options. Whether they chose to go out to eat or stay in, I had detailed instructions. I even included a list of foods with their carb counts and a corresponding chart that indicated how much insulin was needed. I know it sounds crazy, but I needed to set them up for success so they could enjoy time with the kids, and the kids could relax, knowing there was a plan in place for every meal and nighttime lows or highs.

Day one, we were sitting in the airport waiting for our flight, and my mom called to say Jackson was going low. I said, based on his numbers, you can give him a few grapes, which should pick him up. Well, 30 minutes went by, and she called again. I was watching his numbers closely and asked, "How many grapes did you give him?"

She said, "I only gave him one."

I said, "It's okay, Mom. You can give him three grapes."

At that point, I had to step back and remind myself that she was probably a bit nervous and didn't want him to go too high, especially on day one. So, I walked her through my chart again and let her take it from there. It was one of the hardest things I had ever done, but I knew I needed to do it. He was in great hands.

So, off to Napa we went. By day three, I slept through the night and didn't even wake up. I couldn't believe it. It was the most amazing sleep, and I woke up feeling so energized. The kids had sent pictures of all their activities and arts and crafts projects. My husband and I were having such a lovely time with our friends, visiting vineyards, exploring charming small towns, and shopping. This trip was a true spark of joy for my husband and I to reconnect and have time for us while the kids had so much fun with my parents.

> By day three, I slept through the night and didn't even wake up. I couldn't believe it. It was the most amazing sleep, and I woke up feeling so energized.

Then day five came around, and we started our journey back to San Francisco to hop on our flight. I got a frantic call from my mom, who sounded terrible—raspy voice and congested. She had been sick for the last three days and hadn't told me because she didn't want to worry me. Unfortunately, this had trickled to Jackson. That morning, his blood sugar had dropped into the 40s, which is *really low*, and he was refusing to eat anything. This can be very scary, as he would need to go to the hospital if his blood sugar continued to go down and wouldn't eat. My heart and stomach dropped. I was at least a nine-hour flight away from him and couldn't be there to help.

I was so nervous but had to remind myself to stay calm and try to talk Jackson into eating something. My mom put him on the phone, and I explained to him that he needed to eat, even though he didn't want to. His body needed it. He was crying so hard, and all I could do was comfort him through the phone, letting him know it would be okay and that he needed to eat so he would start feeling better. I started giving him every option in the book: apples, fruit bar, watermelon, strawberries—I even went as far as offering him skittles, M&Ms, sour patch kids, which we rarely eat. He didn't budge, which made me even more nervous. My sweet Marlee Kate finally got him to eat something. Grapes for the win!

Let me tell you, that was the longest flight I have ever been on. It was so hard, not being able to see his numbers and call my parents. But I had to trust and know he was in good hands. If you're wondering whether my binder covered this situation, the answer is "no." I would have never expected this to happen. But my parents and Marlee Kate were rockstars and kept him level until we landed and got back to their house.

♡ Advice:

When you travel away for the first time, just remember that you can't plan for everything. No matter how detailed your preparations are, unexpected things will come up, and you'll have to guide whoever is helping you through those moments. It's part of the journey, and a learning experience, not only for us, but also for those amazing people who step in to support us.

When my mom called, frantic and sick, with Jackson's blood sugar dangerously low, I was miles away, helpless and scared. I realized then that I couldn't control everything, no matter how hard I tried. But I also learned to trust and rely on the support around me. My daughter, Marlee Kate, stepped up in ways I hadn't expected, proving just how resilient and resourceful our loved ones can be.

Take the time to accept help when it's offered. I'd do it all over again, despite the chaos and anxiety, because those experiences teach us and strengthen our bonds. Everything happens for a reason, and there's always a silver lining. For me, it was seeing how my family could come together, even in my absence. So embrace the adventure, trust in your support system, and remember to find the positives in every situation. If you would like more information on the guide that I used please see my resource section that will give you an outline to start with.

Tips:

- My parents felt it was very helpful to have a ratio breakdown for each of the meals and options.
- Have the quick guide printed and laminated for quick reference.

10

EDUCATION ESSENTIALS: NAVIGATING SCHOOL WITH TYPE 1 DIABETES

Colorful Starbursts, Skittles, Peanut M&Ms, or Dum-Dums were often handed out for doing a great job on a test, helping a teacher, or answering a trivia question correctly when I was in school. I remember in elementary school, going to a local ice cream shop, "Chilly Jillys," for a free ice cream or slushie as a big reward for the class. These moments were such highlights for me and my classmates.

As I reflect on these memories, I wonder why we needed these sugary rewards. Did they really motivate us to do better on a test or strive for better grades? Perhaps, at times, they did encourage us to study harder or push ourselves. But why did the rewards have to revolve around sugar—and not natural sugar from fruit, but manufactured sugar stripped of all its nutrients and offering no real nutritional value?

It's well known that processed sugar triggers the release of dopamine in the brain's reward center, the VTA. This is the same pathway activated by addictive drugs such as cocaine and heroin. So, I ask myself, why do we need this in school as a reward? That's a bigger topic for a different day!

So, why am I talking about this? When my daughter was in school, I didn't worry too much about the rewards given out at school, or anywhere, because we followed the 80/20 rule, keeping candy as an occasional treat. But when Jackson started school as a diabetic, my perspective changed entirely. I realized I needed to be proactive, just as mothers or caregivers are when their child has an allergy to peanuts, dairy, or gluten. I needed to ensure Jackson and the school were set up for success. So, below, I have outlined my approach when it comes to school, which extends far beyond sugar intake.

Approaching School: Setting Up for Success

There are many things to consider and prepare for to ensure your child is set up for success. Every school operates a little differently, but here is some guidance I can offer you to help your child navigate going back to school or attending for the first time.

Guidance Counselor/Principal

Whether your child is returning to school after a diagnosis or attending for the first time, set up a meeting with the guidance counselor and principal, if possible. If you are unable to meet with them in person, offer to call or have a Zoom meeting. Once you have secured this, you will need to be prepared with a list of questions to facilitate the conversation. This will allow for you to plan for your child's needs while ensuring you are respectful of their time. Below are some suggestions; I also have them listed in my resource section.

- What medical forms are required before my child returns or attends school?
- What medical forms are required annually?

- How do we set up a Medical 504 plan? (This may vary by state.)

    Include exceptions for unlimited bathroom access, unlimited water, testing guidelines to ensure your child is in range before tests (because high or low blood sugar affects brain function), and access to their phone if they have a CGM.

- Do you currently have any students with type 1 diabetes? If so, do you have any recommendations for us involving processes you currently use that work really well?
- May I meet with his/her teacher before my child returns to school?
- Will all staff that interact with my child be trained to use emergency glucagon and recognize signs of low or high blood sugar?
- May I meet with the nurse to discuss my child's specific needs?
- What can I do to help make this process smoother?

♡ Advice from a Principal:

What steps do you recommend parents take to ensure their child feels comfortable and confident about returning to school?

Communicate with the school before the school year begins. The more information that is shared and understood, the better. Share information regarding your child's medical history, current medical status, family medical preferences, and steps to take if medical needs arise at school. When discussing "medical needs" or status changes that require school action, it is beneficial to describe what medical needs look like when your child is experiencing them and how to respond. Each child is unique. Clarity is key.

At first, you may feel like an "educator" on the team when it comes to helping the school team understand what wellness for your child looks like. You know your child best and you are likely the expert on the uniquenesses of your child's medical condition. The school team can learn from you, so consider sharing resources that consolidate information in the form of lists or quick references that help guide discussions to ensure your child's wellness.

Ask questions to ensure connection with the right people. Medical/health plans or formal plans, such as a 504, at school require collaborative partnership. Asking questions such as:

- Does your school have a Multi-Tiered System of Support?
- Who implements school medical or healthcare plans for your school?
- Who is the school 504 coordinator?
- Can we meet before school starts to ensure my child's plan is complete and shared with the appropriate members of the school team?

During the meeting, aim for clarity. It may be helpful to share questions with the school personnel who are setting up the meeting so they have time to consider and answer your questions. This is especially true when students are entering a new school who are not familiar with them or if a team member is new (principal, school nurse, secretary, etc).

As you collaborate to make the plan, include:

- How and when medical supplies and resources are delivered to the school with appropriate documentation.
- Is there a clinic or school nurse onsite daily?
- Who oversees the school clinic if the school nurse is absent or tending to another building?
- Who do I contact if I have questions, concerns, or adaptations to the plan? Share contacts.

- Who do I contact during the school day if there is a medical need, issue, or emergency? Share contacts.
- Who will make sure all staff who are invested in my child's education are aware of the plan?
- In the event of a predicted or unpredicted change in the school day, how will my child access their medical supplies if needed? (substitute teacher, field trips, drills, evacuations, field day, etc.)
- Talk through potential outlier incidents. For example, discuss the appropriate actions in the event that the child does not or cannot comply with the plan.

Include the student in the plan in ways that are age appropriate. It is of utmost priority to ensure students feel they are a valued member of their school team. When students have medical or health needs, it is important they are aware and feel safe. In order to ensure this, parents and teachers may work together to debrief and reassure the child about the steps that are involved in the healthcare plan. As the child gets older, he or she may provide input to the parent and the parent may represent that input to the meeting. Other times, the child may participate in the meeting and start to advocate for their healthcare plan. It may be appropriate for them to have voice and choice in how the plan operates within the school day, while functioning within the bounds of school policy, family preferences, and medical recommendations.

Introduce your child to his or her school team. Providing an opportunity for a child to meet his or her team is essential for both the student and the team. This also encourages familiarity and trust. Back to School Night or a quick appointment can serve as modalities to set up a meet and greet. After meeting and greeting the team members, it may be wise to walk from the child's classroom to the clinic, or other necessary places within the school, so they are comfortable with routines as well.

How can parents work with the school to develop a plan that addresses their child's specific needs, such as an Individualized Healthcare Plan (IHP) or 504 Plan?

Being proactive in information sharing is imperative. Understanding the uniquenesses and accommodations required in order for a child to function at their full potential should always be the goal. The plan should include, but not be limited to:

- Medical documentation
- Impact of medical condition (diabetes)
- Treatment plan and school-based medical administration
- Accommodations / Testing accommodations
- Emergency action

Make sure you know who is responsible for initiating, implementing, and monitoring the plan.

What type of information or training should parents provide to teachers and school staff to ensure everyone is knowledgeable about managing their child's diabetes?

Providing medical documentation, resources, and even helpful links regarding your child's diabetes, treatment/wellness routines, and medical needs can be helpful. The staff member overseeing the student's Individual Healthcare/Medical Plan or other formal plan will be a key person in helping maintain the team's understanding and implementation of the plan.

It is important that there is a discussion about information sharing, as schools are held to standards that uphold confidentiality, such as the Family Education Rights and Privacy Act (FERPA).

You may ask what kind of training the school provides their staff.

How should parents prepare their child to communicate with teachers and peers about their condition, if necessary?

This is a great question. Empowering the student is essential as they learn to advocate for their wellness. First, consider what is important to your child to share and what is important to keep private. Jot down those preferences. I would recommend sharing that with the team so they are also aware. I would suggest working on three types of communication.

1. How do I talk about my diabetes if/when I am ready with my teachers and my peers? This is important from a safety perspective.
2. How do I ask for help when I am not feeling well?
3. How do I respond to peers? Peer-related questions are likely those that are hardest to prepare for, because when kids are curious, they typically just ask. Work with your child to have pre-planned answers for questions that could arise when kids are curious, like:
   - Why are you leaving class?
   - Why do you see the nurse?
   - Why do you get snacks that we don't get?
   - Why can't you eat that?
   - Why do you have a phone or monitoring device?

What advice would you give to parents about maintaining open communication with the school regarding their child's health and any changes in their diabetes management?

Open communication is key. Proactive communication regarding the initial development of the plan often gets the most attention. However, I have learned that the maintenance of communication is incredibly essential. When there are day-to-day changes that need moderated or needed adjustments to the plan, call the point person at the school immediately. Information is power.

Make sure all contact information is up to date. If there are changes to contact information or changes in availability, please make sure the school team knows.

Provide feedback. When adjustments or concerns arise, be open- and solution-minded until the issue is resolved. Additionally, when you are pleased with the team's response, care, and implementation of the plan, let them know. School personnel aim to do what is best for each and every student each and every day, and there is often a vacuum of feedback. As a school administrator, I want to know when my team performs and when they do not. Mrs. Kill has shown our team the value of validation and, because she is an engaged team player, who leads with a positive attitude in advocacy for her son, equips us with the information and resources necessary to care for her son, provides feedback when changes need to occur, and never fails to show her appreciation.

Written by Ashley Thompson

Teacher

Connecting with the teacher is so important as well. In my experience, teachers are eager to help your child succeed. I've met with Jackson's last four teachers prior to school starting so I could get to know them, and they could get to know me. This was really important to me, as I knew my kiddo would be with them almost eight hours each day and I wanted to ensure they understood his background, personality, what he does when his blood sugar is high, and signs to look out for when his blood sugar is low. I also provided a small emergency kit for lockdowns or other emergencies that may come up. Additionally, I offered to replace sugary treats with alternatives like pencils, glow sticks, or stickers. These can be found inexpensively at dollar stores, or online, in bulk. While I don't aim to eliminate all treats, providing alternatives supports a healthier reward system if the teacher is open to it.

Topics to Discuss:

- It is important to provide an overview of your child's diagnosis to ensure the teacher and staff understand the condition and how it may affect their day-to-day activities.
- Share details about your child's personality and how they manage their condition. For example, are they more private and prefer to keep it to themselves, or are they open and would appreciate a book about type 1 diabetes being read to the class to inform their peers?
- Make sure the teacher knows how to recognize and respond to your child's blood sugar highs and lows, as this is crucial for their safety and well-being.
- Inform the teacher about any specific dietary restrictions that your child needs to follow so they can support appropriate snack and meal choices.
- Suggest alternatives to sugary rewards that can be given in the classroom, in case the teacher uses food as a motivator.
- Explain the best routine for your child to go to the nurse's office for blood sugar checks or insulin, especially during lunch or when they experience high or low blood sugar. For instance, Jackson's phone vibrates as a reminder to go to the nurse's office for his lunch insulin 10 minutes before eating, which helps the insulin work before he begins his meal.
- Lastly, remind the gym teacher about any special considerations regarding physical activity, ensuring they fully understand the impact of exercise on your child's blood sugar and how to handle it during class.

I make a kit for each of the classrooms or areas in which he will be in for the day (i.e gym, art, music, homeroom classroom); that way, in the event something happens, everyone has a kit to keep him safe.

Items that we have in our emergency kit:

- Glucose tablets or gel
- Quick-acting sugar (i.e. juice boxes, honey packets, honey suckers)
- Contact information for myself, my husband, and healthcare providers
- Any supplies that might need to be added for a pump
- My outline of the actions to take at each blood sugar level (see my resource section for more information on this outline)

Nurse

Not to scare anyone, but a good friend of mine had a frightening experience when a nurse, thinking she administered 4 units of insulin for lunch, ended up with her child's blood sugar reading as "HIGH," meaning it was well above 400. This caused a lot of panic as the mother tried to understand what went wrong, and the nurse wasn't sure either. The mother waited an hour and then injected a small amount of insulin to start with, assuming the nurse hadn't primed the needle. Sure enough, that was the root cause of the problem.

I share this story to emphasize the importance of ensuring that the nurse and any substitute nurses fully understand the insulin administration process. This is why it is so imperative that you meet with your school nurse either before your child starts school or returns back to school so you can work together in setting up a great plan for everyone to be successful.

♡ Advice from a Nurse:

In speaking with several school nurses across different districts, a common theme emerged: communication is essential. Each nurse emphasized that strong communication, built on trust, honesty, and openness, is crucial to keeping things running smoothly. These qualities create a supportive and collaborative environment that helps ensure the best possible care for each child.

To help make the transition back to school after diagnosis as smooth as possible, see below for key points to consider. By fostering a strong partnership with your school nurse and keeping these points in mind, you can help ensure that your child receives the highest level of care and support during their school day.

Build a Relationship:
- Share an overview of your child's medical history and some of their favorite hobbies and interests. This helps the nurse build a relationship with your child, making them feel more comfortable going to the nurse for injections or corrections.

Daily Routine Review:
- Discuss your daily routine and how you manage your child's insulin needs. This is also a great opportunity to learn from the nurse, who may have valuable insights or ideas based on their experience with other children.

Emergency Protocol:
- Review your emergency protocol and provide the nurse with the type of fast-acting glucagon you use to ensure familiarity. There are several types on the market, so it's important the nurse knows which one your child uses.

Physician Contact Information:

- Provide the nurse with your physician's contact information. In case you are unavailable, the nurse should be able to reach your child's physician for guidance.

Handling Lows and Highs:

- Outline how you handle low and high blood sugar situations, specifying what you prefer to give your child in each scenario. This personalized approach ensures the nurse can provide the best possible care.

Communication:

- Establish a clear communication plan. Effective and consistent communication between you and the school nurse is crucial for harmonizing care and ensuring your child's well-being.

Bus Driver

One area that can often get overlooked is the importance of meeting with the bus driver and coordinator to provide them with the same overview you give to teachers. From my experience, it's crucial to ensure everyone involved in your child's daily routine is well-informed.

During Jackson's first year riding the bus, I organized a training session for our bus driver to equip him with the necessary tools and knowledge on how to handle any potential situations. They were very appreciative of the training. Luckily, we've never had any major emergencies, but there was one stressful moment when Jackson's blood sugar dropped very low.

I was monitoring his numbers on my phone and saw them dropping rapidly. I tried calling Jackson, but he wouldn't pick up. I must have called him about 12 times with no response. In a panic, I decided to drive and flag down the bus to get Jackson. Fortunately, the bus was still in our neighborhood, but it was nerve-wracking knowing his blood sugar was below 40, and he wasn't answering his phone.

After that event, Jackson became more aware and started answering his phone promptly. He didn't want his mom stopping the bus again! Please find below topics to discuss with the bus driver and coordinator of the transportation for the school.

Training Session:
- Organize a training session for the bus driver and coordinator. Provide them with a detailed overview of your child's diagnosis, emergency protocols, and how to use any necessary medical equipment.

Emergency Contact Information:
- Ensure the bus driver has your contact information and your child's physician's contact information.

Emergency Kit:
- Provide an emergency kit that includes fast-acting glucose, a blood glucose meter, and instructions on what to do in case of low or high blood sugar.

Communication Plan:
- Establish a clear communication plan for the bus driver to contact you in case of an emergency.

Regular Updates:
- Regularly update the bus driver on any changes in your child's protocol or management plan.

♡ Advice:

Through all of this, it's important to remember that the receptivity of school leadership can vary depending on the school and its administration. Some schools may be very receptive, while others may not be as accommodating. However, it's crucial to always advocate for your child's needs.

I know that, at times, it can be uncomfortable, but it is so important. For the most part, I've heard very positive responses when parents or caregivers request to meet. The key is to always be respectful of their time and come prepared. Here are a few tips for advocating effectively:

Be Prepared:

- Bring all necessary documentation, including medical records, insulin plans, and emergency protocols.
- Have a clear outline of what you want to discuss and any specific accommodations your child needs.

Respect Their Time:

- Schedule meetings in advance and be punctual.
- Keep the meetings focused and concise to respect the staff's time.

Communicate Clearly:

- Clearly explain your child's diagnosis, needs, and any specific concerns you have.
- Provide examples of how certain accommodations can help your child.

Build Relationships:

- Foster a collaborative relationship with teachers, nurses, and school administrators.

- Share positive updates and express gratitude for their support.

Follow Up:

- After meetings, follow up with an email summarizing the discussion and any agreed-upon actions.
- Regularly check in to ensure that accommodations are being implemented effectively.

By being proactive and prepared, you can ensure that your child receives the support they need at school. Remember, you are your child's best advocate, and your efforts can make a significant difference in their well-being and academic success.

11

JACKSON'S DIAVERSARY: CELEBRATING STRENGTH

I didn't fully grasp the concept of a "diaversary" until I connected with a friend in the diabetes community. She explained to me that a "diaversary" is a term used in the diabetes community to mark the anniversary of a person's diagnosis with diabetes. On this day, individuals reflect on their journey, celebrate their progress, and acknowledge the challenges they've overcome since their diagnosis. It's a time for gratitude and self-reflection, highlighting the resilience and strength of those living with diabetes.

Reflecting on a "diaversary" conjures a complex mix of emotions: sorrow, despair, bafflement, and grief. It took us three years to find any semblance of joy on this day for Jackson. But his fourth "diaversary" shed a new light, sparking a long-awaited joy in our hearts.

During a meal at our beloved eatery, as Jackson's anniversary approached, we pondered on how he might wish to mark the occasion. He fondly reminisced about his hospital stay, which to him felt like Christmas arriving prematurely. Confused, I probed for clarity. He vividly recounted the hospital's treasure trove of toys, the surprise visitor who gifted him a wooden train to paint even in bed, an unheard-of treat at home, and the endless fun with a new Hot Wheels set by the hospital window.

Eagerly, he proposed that we should buy toys for other children at Nationwide Children's Hospital on his "diaversary." And so, with a resounding chorus of approval, our new tradition was born.

> Eagerly, he proposed that we should buy toys for other children at Nationwide Children's Hospital on his "diaversary." And so, with a resounding chorus of approval, our new tradition was born.

On December 22, brimming with anticipation, we set out for Target to transform a day previously shrouded in gloom into one of healing and joy. The store, bustling with pre-Christmas shoppers, could hardly contain my children's excitement. Jackson led the charge, his cart filling with Legos for toddlers and intricate sets for older children, while Marlee Kate carefully chose items suitable for a hospital stay under Jackson's considerate guidance.

Their thoughtfulness filled the cart to the brim, and we made our way to the hospital, emotions in tow. The reality of returning hit me unexpectedly, tears welling up as we walked through those familiar doors. The grateful staff member who greeted us captured the moment, a memento of the kindness my children had spread on the endocrinology floor.

As we departed, Jackson, with maturity beyond his years, expressed a desire to continue this act of benevolence annually. That "diaversary" crystallized a new understanding for us: it took four years to fully grasp the magnitude of Jackson's journey—his daily courage, his endless fluctuations of highs and lows, and the enormity of his heart that thought of others on a day meant to celebrate him.

It was a momentous shift for us all. We had learned, grown, and discovered as a family how to support not only Jackson but countless others navigating similar paths. This "diaversary" marked a new chapter: a journey from hardship to serenity, and from solitude to sharing boundless joy.

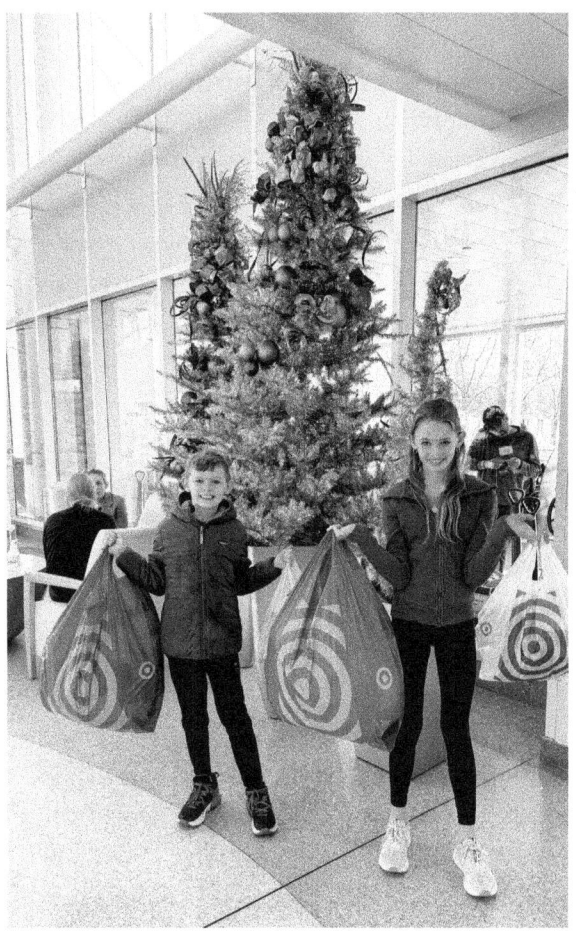

♡ Advice:

This day's meaning is yours to decide, whether you want to celebrate it or not. Trust your heart and choose what feels right for you. Just like it has in our experience, it might evolve over the years, and that's okay. Each person has their own unique journey, and there's no right or wrong way to navigate through it. What matters most is finding the sparks of joy along the way.

Tips:

- Throw a "Hero's Party:" Celebrate your child's courage and perseverance with a superhero-themed party. Encourage guests to dress up as heroes to honor the everyday bravery of living with diabetes.
- Adventure Day: Plan a day filled with your child's favorite activities. Whether it's a trip to the zoo, a movie, or a picnic in the park, let the focus be on fun and celebration.
- Give Back Together: Many kids find joy in helping others. Consider organizing a toy drive or fundraiser for diabetes research or to support other children with chronic illnesses.
- Diabetes Time Capsule: Create a time capsule with items related to your child's diabetes journey. Include blood glucose logs, pictures, a list of achievements over the year, and a letter to their future self.
- Educational Outreach: Sponsor a classroom- or school-wide educational session about diabetes. It empowers your child and raises awareness.
- Custom T-Shirts or Jewelry: Design t-shirts or jewelry with meaningful symbols or slogans that celebrate their journey and resilience.
- Reflection and Goal Setting: Take time to reflect on the past year and set goals for the next. This could include managing levels, trying new foods, or starting new activities.
- Special One-on-One Time: Sometimes, the best celebration is just having some uninterrupted time with a parent. Go out for a meal, take a walk, or engage in a shared hobby.

- Art Project: Encourage your child to express their feelings about their diabetes journey through art, which can be therapeutic and celebratory.
- Donation in Their Name: Make a donation to a diabetes charity or research organization in your child's name to help support the community.
- Plant a Celebration Garden: Plant a tree or a small garden as a living symbol of growth and life, representing your child's strength and growth each year.

12
DISNEY MAGIC: MANAGING TYPE 1 ON THE GO

Disney is often hailed as the happiest place on Earth, a magical destination where children dream of meeting their favorite characters, enjoying thrilling rides, and soaking in the vibrant atmosphere. I never imagined that a place filled with so much joy could also hold a moment of sadness for us. Yet, it happened, and it took us completely by surprise.

Jackson and I were embarking on our first trip together, just the two of us. We had the opportunity to join some dear friends at a conference in Orlando, and as I booked our flights and hotel, a thought struck me: this was the perfect chance to return to Disney. It had been three years since our last visit, and ever since his diagnosis, Jackson had been longing to go back.

I diligently researched all the updated procedures for booking rides. Since we had just one day at Hollywood Studios, I was determined to pack in as many rides as possible. The night before, I meticulously planned our itinerary, prioritizing the rides and experiences to maximize our time. Unfortunately, things didn't quite go as planned. I got up at 7 a.m. to book the Genie+ passes, only to find that everything

Jackson wanted to ride was already booked for the day. *Oh my goodness, what now?* I thought, feeling a mix of disappointment and urgency.

I quickly woke Jackson up and we discussed a few other options. We managed to book alternative rides, but they were all spread out across the park later in the day. Realizing the amount of walking we'd have to do, I decided to pack plenty of "low" snacks.

After navigating three bus rides, we finally arrived at Hollywood Studios. Upon arrival, I noticed the Disability Access Service (DAS) desk. I remembered a parent mentioning it a year ago and thought it wouldn't hurt to check it out. I was immensely grateful I did. The staff was incredibly helpful, quickly setting us up with the service. Thanks to their assistance, Jackson and I were able to jump right onto his first two rides of the day: the Alien Saucers, followed by Smuggler's Run. Jackson's blood sugar started to plummet rapidly, necessitating a quick break amid our Disney adventure. It was an intensely hot day, and the heat only intensified his discomfort. When blood sugar drops, everyone reacts differently, but for Jackson, it meant weak legs and a painful belly, difficult conditions for a young boy who had only enjoyed two rides so far. He looked up at me, exhausted and overwhelmed, and said, "Mom, I just want to go back to the hotel and go to bed."

A flood of emotions washed over me. Was he going to be okay? Was he actually sick? Had I brought enough to adequately raise his blood sugar? Should we just leave? Amidst my swirling thoughts, a gentle breeze brushed past, bringing with it a moment of clarity. I decided we should find a popsicle, a quick, cooling sugar boost, and then sit for about 20 minutes to let his levels stabilize.

I have never been so grateful for a popsicle stand and a nearby seating area in my life. Those 20 minutes felt crucial as I watched him closely. After finishing his popsicle, Jackson's condition improved dramatically; he was back to his cheerful self, ready to take on more rides.

During this time, I had to cancel our ride reservations to manage the situation, but as luck would have it, once Jackson recovered, I checked the app again and discovered an available spot for Slinky Dog Dash, his absolute favorite ride and one that usually has one of the longest wait times. Securing it felt like a small miracle—a spark of joy that lifted both of our spirits.

> ••••••••••••••••••••
> I have never been so grateful for a popsicle stand and a nearby seating area in my life.
> ••••••••••••••••••••

Revitalized, we then ventured into the world of Star Wars with the Rise of the Resistance, and capped our day with Mickey and Minnie's Runaway Railway. It turned out to be a memorable day of resilience, filled with unexpected sparks of joy, a true testament to the magic of Disney and the bond between Jackson and me.

♡ Advice:

If you're planning a trip to Disney or any theme park and you or your child has type 1 diabetes or a disability that qualifies, I highly recommend obtaining the Disability Access Service (DAS) pass. This service was a game-changer for us. Without the DAS pass, we would have struggled to enjoy even a fraction of the attractions. It not only accommodates special needs with less waiting in line but also provides a flexibility that can greatly enhance your experience.

I'm deeply grateful for this service; it played a crucial role in making our day not just manageable but genuinely special. Another practical tip for those managing diabetes or similar conditions is to pre-plan your meal stops. Identify and map out the food stations within the park that offer snacks or meals suitable for your dietary needs and that can help in quickly addressing any blood sugar concerns.

Having a plan for where to find the right kind of food would have made our trip smoother. It's a small preparatory step that can make a big difference, ensuring that you're ready to handle any lows without unnecessary stress. This foresight allows you to focus more on the fun and magic of Disney, ensuring a joyful and carefree visit.

Tips:

- Have lots of low snacks. (i.e. juicy fruits, grapes, oranges, apple juice, gummies etc.)
- Make sure your insulin is protected so it doesn't get hot. There are a couple of options online, including Frio, VIVI cap, and other retailers that can be helpful.
- Plan out where you are going to eat, and just know it could change based on ride availability.
- Breathe, stay calm, and trust your instincts. Maybe breathe again!

13

SUPER SITTERS: TYPE 1 TIPS FOR BABYSITTERS

Everything changed after Jackson was diagnosed. I'll never forget the day my parents insisted my husband and I go out on a date. They practically pushed us out the door, insisting we couldn't come back for at least three hours. I bet you can't guess how many times we checked our phones to see what his blood sugar was… No, I'm not going to share because it's a bit embarrassing. We had a hard time walking away. But looking back, it was the start of us taking baby steps toward getting comfortable with others watching Jackson. It began with quick errands walking through Target, and eventually evolved into real breaks. This was the beginning of a new chapter for us.

> •••••••••••••••••••
>
> We had a hard time walking away. But looking back, it was the start of us taking baby steps toward getting comfortable with others watching Jackson.
>
> •••••••••••••••••••

Those first six months, leaving the kids with my parents now and then, were crucial. They helped us build a foundation for when we felt ready to trust babysitters outside the family. Here's what we learned, as well as the guide we developed to ensure Jackson and Marlee Kate were well taken care of.

In an ideal world, the perfect babysitter would be someone who also has type 1 diabetes and understands its daily management. That would be a home run! But if that's not possible, the next best thing is someone who is attentive and responsible. Once you've found a candidate, it's great to have a trial period where they spend a few hours with you at home to get a feel for your routine.

When you feel they have a good handle on things, start small. Leave the house for a couple of hours and gradually increase the time. I started by dropping Jackson off at daycare for just two hours and sitting in the parking lot, working from my car. Yes, I had to take tiny baby steps, but I promise you, it gets easier. I still keep an eye on his numbers, but I know that will fade with time.

Here's the guide I have posted on our fridge, which I review with anyone watching Jackson to ensure they know what to do in case of an emergency. I have also included this in my resource section.

1. **Emergency Contacts:**
    - Mom: [Your phone number]
    - Dad: [Your husband's phone number]
    - Nearest Hospital: [Hospital phone number and address]

2. **Medical Information:**
    - Diagnosis: [Details]
    - Symptoms to Watch For: [Specific symptoms related to his condition]
    - Insulin Schedule: [Detailed schedule with dosages]
    - Blood Sugar Monitoring: [We use a Sugar Pixel that shows his numbers at all times]

3. **Handling Emergencies:**
   - What to do in case of low blood sugar: [Steps to follow]
   - What to do in case of high blood sugar: [Steps to follow]
   - When to call parents: [Specific situations]

4. **Contact Information:**
   - Local Friend/Relative: [Name and phone number]

5. **Miscellaneous:**
   - Keep the insulin in a cool place at all times.
   - Always have a low snack handy for any activity.
   - Make sure Jackson's phone is always with him (if you have a CGM).

By following this guide, we found peace of mind knowing Jackson was in safe hands and well cared for, allowing us to step out and take much needed breaks.

♡ Advice:

One of the hardest moments for me was leaving Jackson for the first time after his diagnosis. My heart was heavy with worry, and my mind raced with what-ifs. But the support from my parents, the trial runs, and our careful planning all contributed to slowly building my confidence. I'll never forget sitting in that parking lot, watching the minutes tick by, knowing I was just a few steps away if anything went wrong.

Over time, the fear lessened, and the routine became smoother. My husband and I learned to trust the process and the people who cared for Jackson. It wasn't easy, but every small step was a victory. Now, looking back, those initial moments of doubt and anxiety feel like distant memories, replaced by a sense of accomplishment and resilience.

Tips:

- Always trust your intuition when selecting the right person.
- Never feel you are overcommunicating, as it is very serious if your kiddo becomes too high or too low.
- I like to always leave a rough schedule and have snacks ready (if there is a sibling, it is always nice to have the same snacks ready for them as well).
- Stress the importance of how the "EMERGENCY INSULIN BAG" needs to travel with him everywhere. Even if they are just walking to a neighbor's house. I have also included this checklist in my resource section.

    What's in my EMERGENCY INSULIN BAG?
    * Low snacks: honey sticks, honey suckers, fresh juicy fruit, if possible, apple juice
    * Emergency Baqsimi
    * Insulin
    * Phone charger
    * Emergency contacts

14

PARTY PREP:
TYPE 1 BIRTHDAY PLANNING TIPS

Happy birthday! Wait, birthday? What's on the menu? Are parents staying? How am I going to manage taking my child to a seven-year-old's birthday bash without tipping off anyone about his need for snacks or insulin? All the questions raced through my mind.

Leading up to the birthday party, Jackson and I had several conversations. I always feel, in these situations, I would rather be proactive and plan it out, so he can enjoy the party and not have to worry about what he was eating and how much insulin he would need. That is a lot of responsibility to take on for a seven-year-old. This is time for him to have fun with his friends. So, I needed to turn into ninja mom for the day and figure this out quickly.

I first reached out to the mom hosting the birthday party and explained why I was calling so she didn't think I was totally nuts. So, I asked her if she could walk me through what kind of activities she had planned on having, what kind of food she was thinking about having, when they would be serving the food, and, lastly, if she could let me know what kind of cake she was getting and from where. At this point, I know she probably thought I was crazy. But she was incredible and provided me with all the information.

Step one: I determined I couldn't inject insulin before the party because the cake would be at the end of the party.

So I then gave Jackson a few low snacks to put in his pocket just in case. They had planned a few activities I knew would bring down his blood sugar, so I wanted to make sure he had a few things in his pocket he could eat. This allowed him to play all the games and not have to stop because he was too low.

I then followed up and asked Jackson what he wanted to eat. He told me just the cake. Well, if your kiddos are anything like mine, they are always hungry. So, one of my tricks is to feed him a Thanksgiving-type meal before we even head out to a birthday party, so he doesn't feel so incredibly hungry.

I then calculated the amount of carbs in the cake, and I always add a little extra, about 20 carbs, to give myself some flexibility in case he wants something else. If he doesn't, that's fine, because the cake is served last, and I always keep snacks in the car just in case. This extra buffer allows me to avoid saying the dreaded words *"No, you can't."* That's the one phrase that can upset him on any given day.

I then explained to the host that, when we arrived, I would need to give Jackson insulin "10 mins" before they ate cake. So if she could let me know I would greatly appreciate it.

Lastly, I found the bathroom so, when it is time, I can sneak off with Jackson and give him insulin without anyone knowing. Which is how he prefers it.

Of course, it is then so important to take time to relax and let him have *fun* and be a kid!

This was an amazing experience, and not all of them are like this. Some parents just have their kids over to play and then eat cake whenever they feel like it, making it harder to plan. But, at the end of the day, if you and your kiddo work together, it can flow so well. We have had a few parties where the Thanksgiving meal beforehand didn't really fill him, so he was *starving*. I know you, as parents, have *never* heard that. But it is okay if they eat a little more than you had planned and they're hitting a high. It's okay: breathe, calculate, correct, and know this is just a tiny speck in their overall life and their blood sugar history.

♡ Advice:

If you're hosting a party for a child with type 1 diabetes or allergies, it's incredibly helpful to reach out to their parents or caregivers to ensure everyone has a great time. Here's how you can help.

Tips:

- Share details of the planned food menu.
- Provide information about the cake, even if it's homemade. Simply snapping a picture of the recipe and sending it over can be incredibly helpful.
- Discuss the planned activities. Since some children's blood sugar levels can drop quickly, it's important to ensure they have their low snacks readily available.
- As a parent, it's crucial to have a conversation with your child about their food preferences and any dietary restrictions. This ensures that everyone can plan for a successful party. I always wanted Jackson to feel included and not left out.
- Consider offering party gifts for guests that are non-food related. Bouncy balls, bubbles, fidget toys, or stickers are exciting options that avoid potential allergy triggers and are inclusive for all attendees.

15

PLAYDATE PROS: TYPE 1 TIPS FOR FUN

As they grow up, kids always look forward to playdates at each other's houses, and it was no different for Jackson. Those were the days—diving into new adventures, discovering cool toys, and turning living rooms into epic forts made from every pillow and sheet in sight. Those memories are golden, and as a mom, I wanted nothing more than for Jackson to experience that same magic, especially since they mirror my own childhood.

After Jackson was diagnosed and as the world began to emerge from COVID, I felt it was time to reintroduce that slice of normalcy into his life. We started with simple, short visits at our home, managing his diabetes subtly so it wouldn't overshadow his fun. Whether he needed a sugar boost, for which I'd bring out popsicles for all, or if his levels were high, where I'd have him help me with small tasks, everything was designed to keep his condition under wraps but under control. We did things this way until he was ready to let others know why he needed to eat when he was low or why he needed an injection when his numbers were high. This is one of the decisions that I allowed him to make when he was ready.

Taking the step of letting Jackson go to his friends' houses was huge for us. The first time was just a couple of hours at a nearby friend's home. The mom, though new to managing type 1 diabetes, had an incredible heart and was so supportive. Before he went, I filled him up with a hearty meal to stabilize his blood sugar and walked her through everything she might need, from using the insulin in his bag to handling an emergency with a glucagon shot. It's a lot to take in—many parents get that deer-in-headlights look at first—but it's all part of ensuring Jackson's safety.

That playdate was a blast for Jackson. Seeing his joy was a turning point for me; it reassured me that we could do this, that playdates could become a smooth part of our lives. When he befriended a kid whose mom has a medical background, it was like a weight lifted off my shoulders. Knowing she's got a handle on things lets me breathe easier and lets Jackson just be a kid.

♡ Advice:

Leaving your child with someone else for the first time can be daunting; it's like that heart-tugging moment when you leave your baby at daycare for the first day. But with each playdate, you'll learn more about what to share with other parents and what you might keep to yourself to avoid overwhelming them. Each experience helps you find the balance between safety and independence, enabling both you and your child to thrive. As Jackson grows older, he'll start to take more charge of his own care, but until then, it's crucial to educate those around him.

Tips:

- Pre-Playdate Meal: Always have a hearty meal before playdates to prevent immediate hunger.

- Information Sharing: Give a quick overview or a typed guide of essential care points to the hosting parent beforehand—like handling insulin, recognizing highs and lows, and using glucagon. This helps prevent information overload.
- Diabetes Bag Essentials: Make sure the bag includes:

  Insulin (keep out of the sun)

  Needles

  Glucagon

  Snacks for lows (i.e. juicy fruits like grapes or oranges, apple juice, gummies, etc.)

  Glucose meter, test strips, and a finger-stick device

  Emergency contact information
- Pre-Playdate Planning: Jackson and I would discuss food options and insulin management before he goes so he feels prepared and secure in what he would like to do. That way, there is a plan in place. It doesn't mean we don't deviate from that plan from time to time, but we have an idea of what the time at a friend's house might look like.
- Communication: Let the hosting parent know you're just a call away if they need to make any diabetes-related decisions.
- Breathe: Just take a deep breath and take that next step in the journey. There will be lessons learned, but you are just a phone call away, and this will give you and your child so many sparks of joy as you start to trust each other. Make sure you talk to your child after to understand what you could have done differently to make it smoother. Communication is key!

With these strategies, you can help ensure your child has fun and stays safe at the same time. It's all about making these experiences as joyful and worry-free as possible for them.

16

LAKESIDE LAUGHTER: OUR SUMMER ADVENTURE

On the shimmering surface of our beloved lake, a perfect day of boating, surfing, and tubing with family was unfolding like a cherished memory. Laughter echoed across the water, and the sun's warm rays danced on the waves. It was the kind of day that made you forget all your worries—until disaster struck.

In the midst of our fun, Jackson's phone slipped from his hand and vanished into the lake. This wasn't just any phone; it was the critical device that connected to his continuous glucose monitor. Panic set in instantly. The serene lake, which we knew could reach depths of up to 210 feet, became the backdrop for my rising anxiety. Questions flooded my mind: Do I have another device? Will it sync with his current sensor, or will we need a new one? And the passwords, oh my goodness! Do I have them all and are they all updated?

Luckily, our boat's depth finder showed we were at 50 feet deep. We immediately called a diver, hoping he could retrieve the phone. While waiting for him to arrive, I raced Jackson back to my parents' place and pulled out my master tote, which comes with me everywhere. This tote is my lifeline, packed with everything I might need in a diabetes emergency. I began to unpack: the receiver, an old phone, Dexcoms, everything. As I evaluated our options, I decided to pair Jackson's Dexcom device with my daughter's phone to keep the readings consistent. This way, if the diver found the phone, we wouldn't have to go through the hassle of setting up a new one.

An hour later, the diver arrived. He informed us he didn't have much air left from his previous dive and might have to return tomorrow if he couldn't find it today. My anxiety spiked as he geared up and plunged into the lake. Seconds felt like hours. My mind raced with thoughts of what we would do if he couldn't find it. The stakes felt so high.

Finally, the diver resurfaced, clutching the precious phone in his hand. The wave of relief that washed over me was indescribable. Our excitement was palpable, and to our amazement, the phone was still on and working. That diver became our hero, our beacon of hope, and our spark of joy for the week!

> The wave of relief that washed over me was indescribable. Our excitement was palpable, and to our amazement, the phone was still on and working.

Yet, amid the relief and joy, I felt a profound sense of responsibility and a bit of embarrassment. We've been boating here for 25 years; I should have known better than to bring a phone to the water without a floating case. Astonishingly, this wasn't the first time. Two years ago, we lost Jackson's phone in the water. It sank too deep to retrieve and was gone forever. You'd think I'd have learned my lesson. I guess I like to keep things interesting.

Reflecting on the day's events, I couldn't help but feel a mix of gratitude and frustration. Grateful for the diver who saved the day, for my parents' place where I could regroup, and for the master tote that held all our backup supplies. Frustrated with myself for not being more cautious, for putting us in this position again.

This experience was a stark reminder of the unpredictability of life and the importance of being prepared. Since that day, I've bought multiple floating phone cases and scattered them everywhere—one in the boat, one in the car, one in my tote. I've also made sure all our devices are backed up and synced, with passwords securely stored.

♡ Advice:

Despite the initial panic and chaos, the day ended with a sense of triumph. We faced a challenging situation and came through it stronger, more prepared, and with an unforgettable story to tell. It reinforced my belief in the importance of resilience, quick thinking, and the incredible support of family and community. And, most importantly, it reminded me of the love and dedication we pour into caring for Jackson, ensuring his health and happiness no matter what life throws our way.

Tips:

- Online community is very helpful in situations like this, as someone else may have done this same thing. Maybe they didn't lose a phone in a lake, but a pond, pool, or ocean.
- Staying as calm as you can for your little one is so important, because they can read and feel your energy in these moments. I had to collect myself many times to ensure I wasn't making him anxious.

Create a master diabetes tote: This is a well-organized kit that holds all the essential diabetes supplies, making it easy to grab and go for any situation, from daily outings to emergency trips. (**I use a**

Rubbermaid tote with compartments. A sturdy, compartmentalized Rubbermaid tote keeps everything organized and easy to access. The compartments allow you to separate supplies based on function, so you can quickly find what you need.)

- Alcohol wipes: These are essential for sanitizing skin before injections or applying CGM (continuous glucose monitor) sensors, helping to prevent infection.
- Needles for both quick pen and vial: Always have an assortment of needles for insulin delivery, including those for insulin pens and syringes for vials, in case either method is needed.
- Receiver for CGM (with charger): The CGM receiver, which tracks blood sugar levels in real-time, should always be in the tote, along with a charger to ensure it stays powered during long days or outings.
- Low snacks: Keep a variety of snacks that are quick to boost blood sugar levels in case of a low. These could include glucose tabs, juice boxes, or small packs of gummies.
- Over patches: Adhesive over patches to secure the CGM or other devices in place, especially during physical activity or swimming, to ensure they don't come loose.
- Extra CGM: Always have a backup CGM sensor in the tote in case the current one falls off, gets damaged, or malfunctions.
- Adhesive remover: Adhesive removers are important for gently taking off CGM sensors or over patches without irritating the skin or leaving sticky residue.
- Ketosis strips (always double-check expiration date): Keep these strips on hand to test for ketones in the urine, an important indicator of diabetic ketoacidosis (DKA), especially during illness or persistent high blood sugars.
- Finger poke, stick tester, and strips: Even with a CGM, it's essential to have traditional blood sugar testing supplies as a backup. This includes the lancet device (finger poke), glucose meter (stick tester), and extra test strips.

- Sharps container: A small, portable sharps container is necessary for safely disposing of used needles and lancets, reducing the risk of accidental injuries or improper disposal.
- Emergency Glucagon: Always have a glucagon kit or pen for emergency situations when your child's blood sugar drops dangerously low and they are unable to eat or drink. It's a life-saving medication that should be within easy reach.
- Floating device to hold phones: A floating device ensures that phones used to monitor blood sugar or communicate in case of emergency don't sink if dropped into water. This is especially important during activities around pools or lakes.
- Extra phone (old one from six years ago): Keeping a backup phone in the tote is helpful, especially if it's compatible with diabetes management apps or is linked to the CGM. An old phone can serve as a critical backup if the primary phone is lost or damaged.
- Pump (since we currently do not use a pump, I am not sure what supplies would need to be added to this list): If you use an insulin pump, make sure to include pump supplies such as extra cartridges, tubing, and infusion sets. Even though we don't currently use a pump, this would be essential for those who do.

17

BRACES, GUMMIES, AND GLUCOSE: DENTAL TIPS FOR TYPE 1

If you're anything like me, daily flossing might not be at the top of your to-do list, and yes, I often find myself on the receiving end of a lecture from both my hygienist and dentist. They remind me, rightly so, that regular flossing is crucial for maintaining healthy teeth. Now, I see my kids starting to follow in my less-than-stellar dental habits, which has turned me into a bit of a nag about their oral hygiene. I constantly remind them of the importance of not just brushing but also flossing their teeth. It's a battle, but one worth fighting to instill good habits that will ensure their smiles stay healthy long into the future.

Fast forward to our first dentist appointment after Jackson was diagnosed with type 1 diabetes. He was just four years old, and despite the new challenges we faced, he sat quietly and bravely through his teeth cleaning. But when the hygienist asked if we were flossing daily, I hesitated. Truthfully, we weren't managing to floss his teeth every day. "We're doing the best we can," I admitted, feeling a bit guilty. I could almost hear every dentist reading this cringing at our confession.

The hygienist then asked about his eating habits before bed. I explained that he doesn't typically eat late, except on occasions when his blood sugar dips too low during the night. That's when I'd have to give him something quick and sugary, like honey, fruit, or a gummy to stabilize him. Her next question made me pause; she wondered if there was a less sugary alternative that wouldn't linger on his teeth. While I understood her concern about sugar causing decay, I felt stuck—Jackson isn't a fan of juice, and in those urgent moments, we had to use what worked for him.

She suggested brushing his teeth after each late-night feeding. The idea sounded simple, but the reality of it was daunting. Waking a sleeping child several times a night to brush his teeth would disrupt his much-needed rest. The impact on his overall health from losing sleep seemed like too high a price to pay.

This conversation in the dentist's office turned into an eye-opening moment for me. It highlighted a gap in understanding that sometimes exists even among medical professionals about the realities of living with type 1 diabetes. It became clear that I needed to take every opportunity not just to follow medical advice but to educate healthcare providers about what's practical and sustainable for Jackson's daily life.

This experience became a defining moment in our journey. It reminded me that while we strive to manage Jackson's condition as best we can, sometimes we have to make tough choices. I learned that it's okay to prioritize his immediate well-being over perfect dental hygiene if that's what he needs at that moment. And, in those times when we face a choice between disrupting his sleep or letting a couple of cavities develop, I choose his comfort and peace.

♡ Advice:

Reflecting on this, I find a small spark of joy in realizing that every challenge also serves as a lesson. Educating others about Jackson's needs has become just as important as managing his diabetes. It's about making sure he not only survives but thrives, and sometimes, that means embracing the imperfect but necessary choices we make along the way.

Tips:

- It is very important to prioritize a very good dental cleaning for not only our type 1 kiddos, but all kiddos eating today's sugary treats.
- Regarding any suggestions that may come your way, just remember to brainstorm what works best overall.

Orthodontist

If you've ever had braces, you probably remember those long appointments filled with X-rays, endless teeth checks, and what felt like hours of keeping your mouth open. It's quite the ordeal—one that's etched in my memory from my own youth. So, when it came time for Jackson's turn, I thought I was ready. I assumed I knew what we were in for. Oh boy, was I wrong.

We arrived at the orthodontist, and Jackson, just eight years old, bravely sat through his X-rays. The technology they use now is nothing short of amazing compared to what I experienced as a kid. They showed us these incredible 3D images of his face—like peering behind the skin to see everything underneath.

When the orthodontist entered the room, she brought with her the news many kids dread and others cheer for: "It's time to get braces."

Jackson didn't fall into the excited camp.

As we weighed our options, the office manager sat down with us to discuss braces versus Invisalign. She explained how Invisalign trays are easy to remove, less noticeable, and simple to manage—so different from the braces I remembered. "It's easy," she emphasized, and the idea seemed to light up the room.

Jackson turned to me, eyes hopeful, and said, "Let's go with the Invisalign, Mom."

It sounded perfect.

Six weeks after choosing Invisalign, we were back at the orthodontist's for the fitting. The excitement was palpable until the doctor handed us the trays and explained the rules: Jackson was to wear them 24/7, only removing them to eat. I blinked, absorbing the impact of what that meant. Jackson's diabetes means he needs frequent snacks, especially since he's so active and often experiences low blood sugar. Feeding him wasn't just at mealtimes, it was whenever his body demanded, often in the dead of night.

I reassured myself it couldn't be that hard. Yet, reality struck just two days later.

"Jackson, where's your retainer?" I asked, hoping for a simple answer.

"I might have left it at school, Mom? Not sure," he replied.

After a small panic and a call to his school, we retrieved it the next day.

But the challenges didn't stop. The following day, it was the same drill.

"Jackson, where is your retainer?"

This time, he thought it might be in his pants pocket. Indeed, we found it later in the dryer, thankfully still intact. That night, managing his blood sugar was especially tough. He hit four lows, and each time I had to decide whether to wake him to remove the trays and feed him or try something else. By morning, I was exhausted, and so was he.

I called the orthodontist first thing the next morning. I explained that while Invisalign seemed like a manageable option initially, it was proving too burdensome for a child who already had so much to cope with. Managing diabetes at his age was enough; adding this level of responsibility for dental equipment was proving too much. The trays were easy to misplace, difficult to manage during snack times, and added stress during nighttime lows.

The orthodontist was understanding and promised to work with us to find a more suitable solution. Perhaps traditional braces, with less to manage on a minute-by-minute basis, would offer the stability and less hands-on approach we needed.

So, after deciding against Invisalign, we headed back to the orthodontist's office after school to get Jackson's braces fitted. Based on my previous experience when my daughter had hers put on—which was a swift 20-minute affair—I didn't anticipate any complications. I checked his blood sugar before we went in, and he was steady at 88. He had been calm all day without any intense physical activity, so I felt we were in good shape.

However, the situation quickly became more complex than I had expected. The hygienist had already cleaned his teeth and completed what seemed like a myriad of steps to prepare his teeth for the braces. Just as they were about to start applying the brackets, Jackson's sugar levels plummeted to 47. It took me by surprise.

I turned to the hygienist, a mix of apology and urgency in my voice, explaining that I needed to pause the procedure to give Jackson something to eat because his blood sugar had dangerously dropped. Her response was a moment of unexpected relief, she revealed that she was also a type 1 diabetic. Her understanding and compassion in that situation was overwhelming. She not only empathized with our situation but also helped manage it with patience and kindness.

It was a spark of joy in a stressful moment. Her immediate grasp of the situation and her gentle handling of the delay were invaluable. We were so fortunate to have someone who understood firsthand the intricacies of managing diabetes.

♡ Advice:

When visiting the orthodontist, my key piece of advice is to thoroughly understand all the ins and outs of any procedure or dental appliance being recommended. It's crucial to ask numerous questions. Don't hesitate to probe deeper into how each treatment option might impact your child's daily life, especially if managing a condition like diabetes.

This approach ensures that you're not just passively receiving information but actively engaging with it to make the best decisions for your child and your family. Each question helps build a clearer picture and prevents unexpected complications. By understanding every aspect of the proposed treatments, you can confidently decide what's best for your kiddo—and for you.

Tips:

- Detailed Walkthrough: Always ask for a thorough walkthrough of how any dental appliance will function day-to-day. Knowing how it will be installed, maintained, and what adjustments are necessary to fit your child's routine can help avoid surprises.
- Discuss Daily Impact: It's important to discuss how the appliance might affect your child's daily activities, including eating, sports, and especially their health routines. How will

the appliance be cleaned? What are the emergency protocols if it breaks or malfunctions?

- Monitor Blood Sugar Closely: For children managing conditions like diabetes, the stress of dental procedures can affect blood sugar levels. Be extra vigilant during appointments where appliances are fitted or adjusted. Check their levels before, during, and after the visit to ensure they remain stable.
- Plan for Adjustments: Recognize that getting used to a new dental appliance can take time. There might be initial discomfort or changes in eating habits, which could also impact blood sugar levels. Keeping a close eye on these changes will help you adjust care and treatment plans as needed.

18

SEASONAL SHIFTS: INSIGHTS ON BLOOD SUGAR

Have you ever curled up on the couch on a winter evening, watching a movie or having a game night with your family? The kids build tents in the living room with every bed sheet you have, the family pops popcorn, and joy and love fill the room. Here in Ohio, winters can be very cold, and so days of jumping on the trampoline, riding bikes, and swimming come to an end. We then pivot to building with Legos, playing games, watching movies, reading, and doing lots of homework.

As our first winter approached, I started noticing Jackson's blood sugar levels spiking between meals. His ratios for all his meals began to change, and I was worried. Was he sick? Having a growth spurt? Did his insulin go bad? The list of questions running through my head was endless. After about a week, I followed up with our physician, desperate to understand what was happening.

She quickly explained that Jackson was absolutely fine; he just wasn't getting the same amount of exercise he did when it was warm outside. Without this activity, his insulin needs increased. Oh my goodness, by this much? I knew how important exercise was, but holy cow, this was a big jump. I talked to another mother who had to increase her son's long-acting insulin by three units in the winter because of decreased activity.

Determined to find ways to incorporate winter fitness activities, I wanted to keep Jackson's insulin needs the same, if not just a tad higher. Don't get me wrong, it's not bad to increase insulin use, if needed, but incorporating indoor activities is so beneficial in many ways. So I had to get creative. We purchased jump ropes and a basketball game to put in our garage, and cleaned out the garage so they could play in there and be active even when there was snow outside. We also found an indoor trampoline park and an indoor basketball gym to start going to as well. The key is finding what your child enjoys doing and then finding a way you can incorporate it in the winter.

Bring on the spring and nice hot summer. This is when our bikes come out, and Jackson continues racing up and down our street a million times, jumping on the trampoline, and playing in the yard. I love seeing the joy on the kids' faces as they enjoy the outdoors! But I must quickly remind myself to adjust his meals appropriately. This is also a time when he can typically have popsicles without any insulin as well as most fruit. This is the spark of joy in the summer for both of us because he can eat without thinking about coming in for an injection. We are at a point where he will say, "Mom, I am going to jump on the trampoline for 10 minutes and then I am going to have an apple."

He truly understands the impact exercise has on his body and can manage some of this on his own, which, as a mom, just warms my heart.

♡ Advice:

As the seasons change in your life, whether it's literally the weather or your child starting a new sport, it's essential to make gradual adjustments to keep them balanced. Each activity brings different insulin needs, and managing diabetes during these transitions can be challenging but manageable with the right approach. Physical activities can significantly impact blood sugar levels. For example, for Jackson, basketball can cause his blood sugar to drop 50 points within 20 minutes. This rapid burn of energy means we need to find the right snack to fuel him before games or practice.

Tips:

Indoor Winter Activities:

- Small trampoline in the house
- Small basketball hoop in the garage
- Dance parties
- Jump rope in the garage
- Local gym or YMCA to swim or play basketball
- Trampoline parks
- Roller skating
- Indoor obstacle courses

Outdoor Summer Activities:

- Swimming
- Biking
- Roller skating
- Bounce houses
- Climbing on playground equipment
- Sports: any sports that your kiddo enjoys
- Hiking
- Walking in a park: some local parks have activity centers
- Trampoline

Just a reminder—always have diabetes supplies ready, especially during sports and other physical activities. This should include but not be limited to:

- A blood glucose meter or continuous glucose monitor (CGM).
- Low snack, or lots of low snacks.
  * "Juicy Fruits," like grapes, watermelon, oranges
  * Honey Packets—small honey packets under the tongue work fast
  * Honey suckers
  * Applesauce or apple juice
  * Fast-acting glucose (like glucose tablets or juice)

It takes time to find the right balance, but with patience and observation, you can manage it successfully. Keep experimenting with different snacks, insulin adjustments, and activity levels until you find what works best for your child. Remember that what works may change over time as your child grows and their insulin needs evolve.

19

DIABETES MASTERY: THE POWER OF CONSISTENCY

Introduction:

As I searched for answers to my many questions, I discovered the book *Mastering Diabetes* and devoured it in just five days. The science behind improving insulin resistance was fascinating. I couldn't stop. Eager to learn more, I reached out to connect with a coach to support Jackson.

What happened next was remarkable. We started with Jackson needing 1 unit of insulin for 15 carbs, roughly the equivalent of one small apple. But within three days, his breakfast ratio improved to 1 unit for 80 carbs, over five apples' worth. This dramatic shift in blood sugar control was the turning point. We had found our community.

Kylie, our coach, was not only a friend and our biggest cheerleader but also a former pediatric nurse with 18 years of experience. She had worked with many families who had children living with diabetes, which made her guidance even more valuable. Because of her incredible impact on us, I wanted to give her the chance to share something special with you about the power of consistency and how it has helped her husband, who lives with type 1 diabetes, along with so many other families like ours. I cannot thank her enough for all her education and support, and I'm so excited she agreed to share her insights with you.

From Kylie's Experience:

When I entered into my nursing career, I did not know that my path would lead to working with people living with diabetes. I did not expect to become a diabetes expert, through personal and professional experiences, and I certainly didn't expect that I would become a diabetes health coach. I entered my nursing career with an interest in women's and children's health and spent a large majority of my career as a Neonatal Intensive Care Nurse, but often crossed over into pediatrics, and, there, I worked with many families who were newly diagnosed with type 1 diabetes.

All that changed when I met and eventually married a man who was living with type 1 diabetes. When we met and started dating, I don't recall being fazed by diabetes at all—perhaps because I had an understanding of it as a nurse, or perhaps because the way he lived with type 1 was so fascinating. Cyrus had a relationship with type 1 that was so different from anyone else I had experienced. It was very organic and he seemed to perform the routines of living with type 1 with ease. Blood glucose checks, insulin injections, and eating were just so fluid or innate—like the way that you breathe—just another function of his body. What I came to learn, after many years of living with Cyrus and participating in his journey, is that the consistency in his routines, lifestyle consistency, is sort of the "antidote" to diabetes confusion.

Cyrus was diagnosed when he was in his senior year of college, later in the game for a type 1 diagnosis. He was facing graduation and moving into adulthood, searching for his career path. He tells me that he followed the recommendations he got from his doctors to a "T" (and as an engineer, was determined to fix and control his blood glucose). However, within that first year after diagnosis, he was left feeling defeated, depressed, low energy, and had difficulty recovering from exercise or activity, and he didn't know what to do. He eventually found a doctor who would help him with his dietary strategy to optimize his insulin sensitivity, meaning that the insulin that he injected would be the most effective or efficient that it could be in his body. This strategy was a "whole food, plant-based" strategy. After adopting this strategy for less than one month, his insulin use had reduced, his blood glucose had stabilized and become very predictable, he was feeling hopeful and alive, and he was able to move his body. He started going back to the gym, his recovery time reduced, he no longer had crippling leg cramps after a soccer game, in essence, his body was responding to the nutrition in his food.

Cyrus was intrigued: why was it that when he ate the exact opposite way that the doctors recommended, his body started to respond in a positive way? He returned to UC Berkeley to study Nutritional Biochemistry to answer this exact question: why did his cells respond to this dietary approach? And, six years later, he had his answers. He learned everything about how the body functions at the cellular level; he learned about the role of all nutrients: macro, micro, and trace elements; he studied tirelessly to show that dietary influences *are* significant and that we should absolutely care about what we put into our bodies. The answer was very clear… Insulin resistance was the key for understanding blood glucose management.

From his continued education, and his own personal results—it's been over 20 years of following this approach and he's never had an A1C above 6, he uses exactly 24 units of insulin per day (half from long-acting and half from short-acting), and in the time I've known him (12 years, at this point) this hasn't changed much at all. At 44, he also lives with normal cholesterol levels, normal blood pressure, no signs of heart disease, diabetic retinopathy, neuropathy, or other conditions that most people who live with type 1 diabetes have after over 20 years' experience.

He also decided to teach others about this approach (including me). The night we met, he told me "I want to tell the world the truth about diabetes," and I believed him. In 2017, he co-founded a company called Mastering Diabetes: it is a coaching and education program designed to teach and educate people living with any form of diabetes how to reduce and reverse insulin resistance, which is the key to consistent blood glucose management. He co-authored a New York Times best-selling book called *Mastering Diabetes*, which has helped to support and educate thousands of people around the world living with type 1 diabetes, showing them that there *is* power in their hands. And truly, consistency is ***key***.

I have been a coach, investor, and supporter of Mastering Diabetes, our team, and our amazing clients who join us and want to learn how to best take care of their health, particularly when they are living with diabetes. I have always loved working with my type 1 diabetes warriors, especially children—and their families—who are learning how to live with something that can be very confusing and consuming. Being a coach to individuals and families has been a gift, to be able to support people through challenges and find solutions together to overcome them. Whether it's calculating carbohydrates for meals, learning how to adjust insulin dosing, understanding mechanisms of the body to optimize movement and fitness, or so much more, I've truly enjoyed supporting our clients; it's been a highlight of my professional career. Because I love and share a life with someone who is thriving with type 1 diabetes, I wish this for everyone who is not just living with type 1, but who is a partner or parent to someone living with type 1.

As a diabetes coach since 2017, and someone who's worked with hundreds of clients in our program, I have found that the more consistent you can be with daily routines and strategies, the more and more you will optimize blood glucose patterns. These strategies include:

1. Keeping dietary fat to a minimum.
2. Eating meals that contain consistent amounts of carbohydrates for gaining and maintaining weight (especially for growing children).
3. Daily movement, especially first thing in the morning, to utilize glucose.
4. Managing stress.
5. Optimizing sleep.

Working with a coach who is familiar with T1 diabetes blood glucose patterns, carbohydrate:insulin ratio calculation, and understands the daily challenges of blood glucose management is so incredibly valuable. One of the things I have heard over and over again from my clients living with T1 diabetes is that "my diabetes educators never told me this," or "my doctor doesn't teach me these things." Unfortunately, that is a common experience, and that's why coaches are so vital, especially as you are starting down this path. A diabetes coach can help you set up daily strategies for meals, fitness/movement, understand blood glucose patterns from a day-to-day or week-to-week basis, and troubleshoot between doctor's appointments. This will help you build consistency and can help with reducing stress and fear between those appointments. It is also incredibly empowering to learn how to manage the ins and outs of diabetes when everything feels so new and unfamiliar.

There is a lot to process when your child is diagnosed with type 1 diabetes. You are not alone and there are so many amazing resources out there. I hope that we can become one of them for you: children living with T1 diabetes benefit from a role model and someone who is thriving living with T1. I hope my husband and our family can provide hope and be of support to you during this time.

Written by Kylie Buckner, MSN, RN, Diabetes Coach

20
HAPPY HOLIDAYS: NAVIGATING FESTIVE TIMES

Spooky Fun: Halloween with Type 1

If you're anything like me, Halloween presents quite a challenge with all the candy, the blood sugar fluctuations, the excitement, and the unknowns. As much as you try to plan, it's sometimes impossible to account for every variable when it comes to blood sugar levels.

When Jackson was six, he embarked on a journey to outer space as he dressed up as an astronaut for Halloween. While he didn't actually fly into space that night, his blood sugar certainly skyrocketed.

He was bursting with excitement for trick-or-treating, like most kids his age. They couldn't wait to collect candy and visit houses that gave out the coveted large candy bars! Naturally, before any outing, we had our checklist: insulin, low snacks, phone, needles, emergency supplies. We checked everything off and set out.

However, not even 10 minutes into trick-or-treating, Jackson's blood sugar dropped, prompting a snack. Then it dropped again, and again… Oh my goodness, what was happening? Ah, yes, all the running around.

I hadn't anticipated needing so many snacks. So, what did we do? Yes, we resorted to the unknown candy. I wasn't sure what the carb count truly was, so I had to take my best guess, and let's just say I didn't calculate correctly, and he ended up on the moon that night.

But the spark of joy that evening came when Jackson and Marlee Kate decided to donate almost all their candy to a local food pantry, keeping only two Kit Kats for themselves. Who doesn't love a good Kit Kat, after all? This act of kindness filled my heart with happiness. It wasn't because Jackson couldn't have all the candy—he could, but it wasn't ideal for him or anyone else. Their generosity towards those who wouldn't have the opportunity to go trick-or-treating was truly heartwarming.

> But the spark of joy that evening came when Jackson and Marlee Kate decided to donate almost all their candy to a local food pantry, keeping only two Kit Kats for themselves.

We have a good friend who introduced us to the idea of "Ellie the Skeleton," which has become a beloved tradition in their home. Like the Elf on the Shelf in December, Ellie the Skeleton visits them throughout October, bringing a fun and festive touch to their Halloween celebrations. Ellie isn't just a decoration, she takes part in all the Halloween activities, even going trick-or-treating with them.

This year, Ellie took on an even bigger role by helping them manage the mountain of Halloween candy. After a night of trick-or-treating, their daughter decided to give Ellie her candy to take back to "Halloween Town." In return, Ellie left a special surprise for her to discover the next morning. This year, it was an incredible indoor princess tent!

♡ Advice:

Effective communication is crucial, especially in situations like these. It's imperative to listen to your child and understand their needs. You might be surprised to find out that they don't actually want candy; perhaps they would prefer a fidget spinner instead. Open up the dialogue and ask them what brings them the most joy for this holiday, then work together to find a compromise. It's much better than imposing restrictions. Trust me, I've been there too.

Tips:

- Always have double the low snacks, like "juicy fruits," gummies, apple juice, etc.
- Eat before you go trick-or-treating so they are not as tempted to want to eat the candy.
- Have a discussion beforehand about what they would like to do with their candy and offer suggestions.
- Take the candy to a local food pantry.
- Donate to your local school for the staff to enjoy.
- Some dentist offices will offer to buy kids' candy.

Hoppy Days: Easter with Type 1

This holiday, traditionally marked by the eager hunt for colorful eggs—usually filled with a medley of candies like Skittles, Jolly Ranchers, M&Ms, and more—was a vibrant part of my childhood. Our eggs often contained a mix of candy and coins, and each Easter basket brimmed with Cadbury eggs, Peeps, and other sugary delights, alongside a book, bubbles, and a small toy. This delightful tradition continued when we started our own family, until our son Jackson was diagnosed with type 1 diabetes.

This diagnosis prompted my husband and me to reevaluate not just Easter, but all our holiday celebrations. We started questioning why so many of these special days seemed to revolve around food. Did the kids really need 20 mini bags of M&Ms, 10 bags of Skittles, and 15 Kit Kats? This reflection led us to a significant shift in how we celebrated.

We realized that if we looked closely at the reasons behind our celebrations, we could find countless other ways to create joy and make these occasions special. We began focusing on non-food rewards and traditions that could bring just as much happiness without centering on sweets.

> These changes were about more than just adapting to a medical condition; they were about shifting our focus from consuming to engaging. Each item was chosen to encourage play, creativity, and family time—elements that create lasting memories.

My husband and I opted for a refreshing twist on the traditional Easter egg hunt for our kids. Instead of the usual cascade of candies, we filled the eggs with coins and stickers—simple, fun. For the Easter baskets, we went even further in our creative reinvention. We included board games and books, sure to spark joy and ignite the imagination. An umbrella, perhaps an odd choice at first glance, promised fun rainy day walks and a bit of whimsy. Water balloons, kites, and sidewalk chalk rounded out the basket, perfect for hours of outdoor fun and creativity.

These changes were about more than just adapting to a medical condition; they were about shifting our focus from consuming to engaging. Each item was chosen to encourage play, creativity, and family time—elements that create lasting memories. This new approach to holiday celebrations has brought unexpected joy and excitement, highlighting that the spirit of an occasion doesn't have to be tied to traditional expectations but can be crafted around what truly matters to us as a family.

♡ Advice:

If your family celebrates Easter or any holiday that traditionally revolves heavily around food, it might be time to think outside the box for ways to create lasting memories and sparks of joy. Whether it's through coloring books, a new basketball, bubbles, kites, or family board games, the possibilities for fun are endless and don't need to break the bank.

Consider focusing on activities that bring your family together, encouraging play, creativity, and togetherness. These gifts and activities can replace the usual emphasis on food with experiences that everyone will remember for years to come. This shift not only makes the holiday unique, but also healthier, especially for families managing dietary restrictions or health concerns. By reimagining your celebrations in this way, you can craft holidays that are joyful, inclusive, and filled with fun, not just food.

Tips:

- Going to a dollar store with bins in the front that are always discounted is a great start.
- If your kiddo absolutely loves a certain candy, it is still fun to include it as a special treat.

Christmas to Remember

Our first Christmas together post-diagnosis was a day to remember, and not just because it was December 24. We had just come home from the hospital, our daughter was under the weather, and my family was off to Christmas Eve mass. So, we decided to stay home, cozy up, and watch movies as a family. It was a bittersweet evening, full of relief to be home, but also filled with nerves as we checked Jackson's blood sugar every hour to ensure everything was alright.

Christmas morning came with the usual excitement of presents and festive joy. Jackson was bouncing off the walls with anticipation, while Marlee Kate, still not feeling her best, preferred to lounge on the couch. I found myself longing for the chaos of a "perfect" Christmas morning—everyone up, excited, and ready to visit family. Instead, I was charting Jackson's blood sugar readings, documenting his food intake, and researching the best foods for a diabetic diet. In hindsight, my obsessive Googling could have taken a backseat!

Amidst all this, my husband and Jackson were having a blast playing games and building Legos. I had to pause and reframe my perspective. This quiet, imperfect moment was exactly what we needed. It wasn't about the ideal Christmas I had in my head, but about being together, supporting each other, and finding joy in simply being a family.

That day, I realized that holidays aren't about the food, the candy, the bustling family visits, or even the presents. They're about being present with the people we love, sharing time together without the burden of expectations. We don't all celebrate the same holidays, and that's okay. What matters most is the love, care, and compassion we share with each other.

So, here's to embracing the unexpected, finding joy in the simple moments, and celebrating the true spirit of being together.

Tips:

- Ideas on what to bring or serve: there are so many ideas on social media. I typically will go to Pinterest for super creative ideas on how to make fruit fun or minimalist baking ideas for main dishes and sides!

- We love bringing dishes to our holiday gatherings that align with our way of eating, but we always make sure to offer something for everyone to enjoy. It's important to have a variety of options while also maintaining consistency for Jackson's diabetes management.

CONCLUSION

When I first started this journey, I never imagined joy could be part of it. In those early days, all I could feel was heartache, desperation, and sadness as I learned how to inject insulin and count carbs, woke up in the middle of the night to handle low blood sugar, and figured out how to balance highs and lows. Even something as simple as finger-poking to get accurate readings felt overwhelming.

But here's the beautiful part: what once seemed impossible can transform into something powerful. With the right knowledge and tools, and a supportive community, you can face each milestone with confidence. From getting your child ready for school, to navigating that first endocrinologist appointment, or even planning your first vacation, you're never truly alone. There's an entire community of people who understand what you're going through. And, over time, you'll realize that the love you have for your child is greater than any challenge diabetes throws your way. Stay strong, because you are far more powerful than you realize.

I wish you all the best on this journey. Who knows? Maybe one day our paths will cross, and we'll have the opportunity to meet. Until then, let's walk this wild and crazy journey together. Allow love to drive you to keep learning, adapting, and thriving. With love, we find strength and even joy amidst the challenges we face. You are going to shine and be absolutely amazing!

APPENDICES

Diabetes Decoded: Understanding the Diagnosis

I'll break down what type 1 diabetes really is and how it differs from type 2. I'll also dive into the long list of questions I was flooded with in the beginning, as well as some I still get asked today.

Sitting in the hospital, my mind was racing with questions and fears. What exactly is type 1 diabetes? How did Jackson end up with this? Was it something he was exposed to? Is there a cure? Did I eat the wrong thing during pregnancy? Had I somehow fed him the wrong foods when he was little, weakening his immune system? All these thoughts swirled in my head, each one more overwhelming than the last.

Fast forward four years, and while we've learned and continue to learn how to navigate this new journey, the questions from others never stop. Parents, friends, kids, neighbors—anyone who sees Jackson's Dexcom device—ask, "What is type 1 diabetes? Will he ever grow out of it?"

The answer, currently, is no—he will not grow out of it. This is a disease that does not have a cure yet. I say "yet" because I have a good feeling that there will be a cure. We have too many brilliant people in this world today to not find a cure for type 1 diabetes.

What Causes Type 1 Diabetes?

You might wonder, what causes this to happen? The exact cause of type 1 diabetes is still being studied, but several theories exist. One theory suggests that a virus may trigger an autoimmune response that destroys the insulin-producing beta cells in the pancreas. While the cause is not fully understood, it is clear that, without insulin, neither humans nor animals can survive, as it is essential for regulating blood sugar and allowing cells to use glucose for energy.

How Insulin Works in the Body

So how does this work in the body? As you eat, your pancreas produces both digestive enzymes (to help break down food) and the hormone insulin. Insulin is crucial for regulating blood glucose levels by facilitating the absorption of glucose into your cells, particularly in muscles, fat, and the liver. After a meal, rising blood glucose signals the pancreas to release more insulin, allowing your cells to take in glucose. Once glucose levels in the blood return to normal, insulin production decreases. This process helps maintain balanced blood sugar levels.

For people living with type 1 diabetes, the pancreas does not produce insulin at all, so when they eat a meal, the body cannot release insulin naturally. They must manually calculate the carbohydrates in their meal and inject insulin to match it. They may need to wait around 10-15 minutes for the insulin to start working before eating. This timing helps ensure that the insulin is available to meet the glucose from the food, allowing it to be transported into the cells for energy.

Common Questions about Type 1 Diabetes

Can you eat sugar? Yes, people with type 1 diabetes can eat sugar, but they must account for it by adjusting their insulin. While natural sugars from fruits are part of a healthy diet, both natural and processed sugars need to be managed to avoid blood sugar spikes.

Do you need to eat low carb? No, you are not limited to a low-carb diet, but many people find it easier to manage their blood sugar by moderating carb intake. The key is ensuring you are eating nutrient-dense foods that provide your body with energy.

Is this an illness? Yes, type 1 diabetes is both an autoimmune disease and a chronic illness that requires lifelong management.

Can you eat fruit? Absolutely, you can eat fruit, but like all carbohydrates, you need to manage it with insulin to keep your blood sugar in check.

What is a CGM? A Continuous Glucose Monitor (CGM) is a device that tracks your blood glucose levels throughout the day and night by measuring glucose in the interstitial fluid just beneath the skin. Unlike traditional glucose meters, which require finger stick tests, a CGM provides real-time glucose data and reduces the need for frequent fingersticks.

What is a pump? An insulin pump is a small, wearable device that delivers insulin through a thin tube inserted under the skin. It provides both basal insulin (steady, continuous doses) and bolus insulin (for meals), helping individuals with type 1 diabetes manage their blood sugar levels more precisely.

Will you grow out of this? No, type 1 diabetes is a lifelong condition. You will not grow out of it, as the body permanently loses the ability to produce insulin.

How many injections do you have to take a day? The number of injections varies from person to person, depending on their meals and blood sugar levels. Many people take 4-5 injections a day, but this can vary, with some taking more on certain days.

Do you have to wear a Continuous Glucose Monitor? No, wearing a CGM is not mandatory. It is up to the individual based on their preferences and lifestyle. Some prefer using traditional glucose meters, while others opt for continuous tracking.

Do you have to wear a pump? No, using an insulin pump is also optional. People can choose between injections and pumps, depending on what works best for their diabetes management and lifestyle.

Are you able to participate in sports? Yes, people with type 1 diabetes can fully participate in physical activities. However, they need to monitor their blood sugar levels closely, as exercise can affect glucose levels.

Can you get double diabetes? Yes, it is possible for people with type 1 diabetes to develop insulin resistance, a condition typical of type 2 diabetes. This is sometimes referred to as "double diabetes" and requires managing both insulin resistance and insulin deficiency.

How do you test for type 1 diabetes? Diagnosis typically involves blood tests that measure fasting glucose levels, A1C, and the presence of autoantibodies that attack insulin-producing cells.

What happens if your blood sugar gets too high? You will need to inject insulin to lower your blood sugar if it becomes too high (hyperglycemia).

What happens if your blood sugar gets too low? If your blood sugar drops too low (hypoglycemia), you should consume fast-acting carbohydrates, like juice or glucose tablets, to quickly raise your levels to a safe range.

What is DKA?

Diabetic Ketoacidosis (DKA) is a dangerous complication of type 1 diabetes where the body breaks down fats too quickly, leading to a buildup of acidic ketones in the blood. This requires emergency treatment with fluids, electrolytes, and insulin.

What is the honeymoon phase in type 1 diabetes? The honeymoon phase occurs shortly after diagnosis when the pancreas is still producing some insulin, leading to reduced insulin needs. This phase can last from weeks to up to a year.

How often do you see an endocrinologist? Typically, individuals with type 1 diabetes see an endocrinologist every three to six months for regular check-ups and adjustments to their treatment.

Are all foods created equal? No, different foods have varying impacts on blood sugar. Foods high in carbohydrates, especially refined sugars, will raise blood sugar more quickly and need careful management with insulin.

What is the difference between Type 1 and Type 2 Diabetes

Type 1 Diabetes

Definition: Type 1 diabetes is an autoimmune disorder in which the immune system mistakenly attacks and destroys the insulin-producing beta cells in the pancreas. As a result, the body produces little to no insulin.

Characteristics:

- Usually diagnosed in children and young adults, but can develop at any age.
- Requires lifelong insulin therapy to regulate blood sugar.

- Symptoms often appear suddenly and include excessive thirst, frequent urination, unintended weight loss, and fatigue.
- Management: Treatment involves daily insulin injections or the use of an insulin pump, continuous glucose monitoring (CGM), a healthy diet, and regular exercise to maintain stable blood glucose levels.

Type 2 Diabetes

Definition: Type 2 diabetes is a metabolic disorder where the body becomes resistant to insulin or doesn't produce enough insulin to maintain normal blood sugar levels. It leads to elevated blood glucose over time.

Characteristics:

- More common in adults over 45 but is now increasingly seen in younger individuals, including children and adolescents.
- Strongly associated with lifestyle factors like obesity, lack of physical activity, and genetic predisposition.
- Symptoms develop gradually and may include increased thirst, frequent urination, constant hunger, fatigue, and blurred vision.
- Management: Primarily managed through lifestyle modifications, such as a balanced diet, regular physical activity, and weight management. Medications (oral or injectable) may be prescribed, and in some cases, insulin therapy is needed.

Key Differences:

Onset: Type 1 is typically diagnosed in childhood or early adulthood, while type 2 usually develops later in life but is increasingly being diagnosed in younger people.

Cause: Type 1 is an autoimmune condition, whereas type 2 is largely influenced by lifestyle and genetic factors.

Insulin: People with type 1 require insulin for life, while type 2 can often be managed with lifestyle changes and oral medications, though insulin may be needed later.

Diabetes Dictionary: Your Go-to Glossary

Endocrinologists monitor several key markers in patients with type 1 diabetes to manage the condition effectively and prevent complications. Below are the most important markers and why they are closely watched:

Hemoglobin A1c (HbA1c)

What it is: A measure of average blood glucose levels over the past 2-3 months.

Why it's important: HbA1c gives an overall picture of long-term diabetes control. Lowering HbA1c reduces the risk of complications like neuropathy, retinopathy, and cardiovascular disease.

Target range: Typically at or below 7.5% per the American Diabetes Association (ADA), though this can vary based on individual factors.

Blood Glucose Levels

What it is: Regular monitoring of daily blood sugar levels using a glucometer or continuous glucose monitor (CGM).

Why it's important: Daily glucose readings help in adjusting insulin doses, diet, and activity levels to avoid hyperglycemia (high blood sugar) and hypoglycemia (low blood sugar).

Blood Pressure

What it is: Measurement of the pressure exerted by blood against artery walls.

Why it's important: High blood pressure increases the risk of cardiovascular disease and kidney problems, both common complications in diabetes.

Lipid Profile

What it is: A test measuring cholesterol and triglyceride levels in the blood.

Why it's important: Managing lipid levels is key to reducing cardiovascular risk, which is higher in people with diabetes.

Kidney Function Tests

What it is: Includes tests such as serum creatinine, blood urea nitrogen (BUN), and urine albumin-to-creatinine ratio.

Why it's important: Early detection of kidney damage (diabetic nephropathy) can allow for interventions that slow its progression.

Eye Exam

What it is: A comprehensive eye exam, including dilating the pupils, to detect signs of diabetic retinopathy.

Why it's important: Retinopathy, if left untreated, can lead to blindness. Regular exams help with early detection and treatment.

Foot Exam

What it is: A physical exam to check for neuropathy, ulcers, or infections.

Why it's important: Diabetes can cause nerve damage and poor circulation, increasing the risk of foot ulcers and infection. Early detection can prevent serious complications like amputation.

C-Peptide Test

What it is: A test that measures C-peptide, which indicates how much insulin the pancreas is producing.

Why it's important: This test helps differentiate between type 1 and type 2 diabetes and can give insight into remaining beta-cell function.

Autoantibody Test

What it is: Tests for specific antibodies that attack insulin-producing beta cells.

Why it's important: It confirms the diagnosis of Type 1 diabetes and can help predict its onset in individuals at risk.

Conclusion:

The tests and markers outlined here play a crucial role in developing personalized treatment plans for type 1 diabetes. By regularly monitoring these indicators, healthcare providers can help prevent complications and ensure optimal health outcomes.

This chapter references credible sources such as the American Diabetes Association, National Institute of Diabetes, and Mayo Clinic to provide accurate and up-to-date information on diabetes management.

Diabetes Unplugged: Back to Basics

Remember the days of typewriters? Some of us can still hear the click-clack of those clunky keys. Then came computers, transforming the way we write with spell check, synonyms, and even the ability to rewrite entire papers at the click of a button. Today, we've become accustomed to the conveniences of modern technology. But when things don't go as planned, sometimes we need to go back to basics—like writing a handwritten letter or dusting off that old typewriter.

The same can be said for diabetes management. We've come a long way from finger pokes and manual injections to advanced technology like continuous glucose monitors (CGMs) and insulin pumps, which have revolutionized how people manage their diabetes. For some, even a finger poke might seem outdated compared to today's tech!

The diabetes community has seen extraordinary leaps in technology over the past decade. These tools aren't just gadgets—they're game-changers, helping people manage their condition more efficiently. But no matter the advancements, it's essential to stay grounded in the basics, because technology, as great as it is, can sometimes fail—and it always seems to happen at the worst possible time, like just before bedtime.

Imagine this: It's late, your child is almost asleep, and suddenly, a device fails. If your child is anything like mine, they could sleep through anything—even a CGM change without a stir. But for caregivers, these moments cause immediate panic. What's the plan now? How long will we be without the system? These moments truly test our preparedness and resilience.

Just last week, we experienced one of those dreaded outages—right at bedtime. After a quick check on Facebook, I realized we weren't alone. Many others were facing the same issue, frantically trying to troubleshoot and reset their devices. Despite our efforts, our system wouldn't come back online.

While this meant extra vigilance for us, my son Jackson saw it as an opportunity for a "slumber party" downstairs, turning a stressful situation into a little adventure. For us, it meant setting alarms every two hours to manually check his glucose levels. But, truth be told, I checked far more often than the alarms suggested.

♡ Advice:

This experience was a stark reminder of the importance of mastering the basics of diabetes care. Whether it's testing blood sugar manually, counting carbs, or having extra supplies on hand, it's essential to be ready when technology fails.

Tips:

- **Routine Tech Drills:** Every few months, we simulate a tech outage, like a fire drill, for diabetes management. This helps us stay sharp and ensures we can handle things without relying on our devices.
- **Keep Supplies Updated:** Make sure your supplies—like test strips, insulin, and batteries—are always stocked and up-to-date. There's nothing worse than realizing you're out of test strips at 10 p.m. and rushing to the store!
- **Consult Your Endocrinologist:** If you're on a closed-loop system, work with your endocrinologist to create a clear action plan for tech failures. Knowing exactly what steps to take can reduce stress during those critical moments.
- **Lean on Your Community:** Online support groups are invaluable in times of crisis. Whether it's troubleshooting tips or just knowing others are going through the same thing, the community can offer support. Just be cautious—solutions for one device or setup may not work for another, so always check the details for your specific system.

Tech Talk: Diabetes Devices Explained

Our family has chosen not to use an insulin pump at this time. Every family managing diabetes makes choices based on their unique circumstances, and for us, this has worked best. However, technology continues to evolve, and it plays an essential role in diabetes management for many families.

To give you a broader perspective, I've asked a close friend to share her experience using an insulin pump for her daughter. Here's what she had to say:

From a Friend's Experience:

In 2021, after my daughter's diagnosis at age 12, I quickly realized how advanced diabetes technology had become. During her hospital stay, my daughter was adamant that she wanted a Dexcom CGM and a tubeless pump. She said, "I play soccer and don't want tubes while playing or finger pricks on the sidelines." Despite my lack of knowledge, she knew exactly what she wanted.

While we had to wait several months for approval, she eventually received the Dexcom G6 and the Omnipod Dash pump. These tools have made a huge difference in her ability to manage her diabetes while playing sports and living her life as a type 1 diabetic.

That said, technology isn't without its frustrations. We've faced our share of failed sensors, leaky pods, and errors. Still, we're grateful for the advancements that make her life easier. But we've also learned that nothing about type 1 diabetes is "easy," and every hour can bring something different. She has become more resilient and confident in managing her condition.

Diabetes Devices: A Quick Guide

Here's an overview of some of the common diabetes management tools available today:

Continuous Glucose Monitors (CGMs): CGMs track glucose levels in real time, offering alerts for high and low blood sugar.

- Dexcom G6/G7

    Real-time readings every 5 minutes, no finger stick calibration, customizable alerts.

- Freestyle Libre 2

    Scannable sensor, optional alarms, 14-day sensor life.

- Freestyle Libre 3

    Real-time glucose readings, smaller sensor, no scanning needed, 14-day sensor life, real-time alerts for high and low blood sugar.

- Medtronic Guardian Connect

    Predictive alerts, 7-day sensor life, integrates with other Medtronic devices.

Insulin Pumps: Insulin pumps provide continuous insulin delivery, mimicking the body's natural insulin release.

- Omnipod DASH

    Tubeless design, controlled by a handheld device, customizable insulin delivery.

- Tandem tX2

    Slim design, touchscreen interface, integrates with CGM for automated insulin adjustments.

- Medtronic MiniMed 770G

  Hybrid closed-loop system, adjusts insulin based on CGM readings, smartphone compatible.

- Smart Insulin Pens:

  These pens track insulin doses and connect to mobile apps for better diabetes management.

- InPen

  Bluetooth connectivity, gives dose reminders, tracks insulin usage and active insulin.

- NovoPen 6

  Digital display, tracks insulin dose history, integrates with diabetes management apps.

Blood Glucose Meters: Blood glucose meters provide quick, accurate blood sugar readings.

- Accu-Chek Guide

  Bluetooth connectivity, strip ejector, light for testing in the dark.

- OneTouch Verio Reflect

  Personalized insights, Bluetooth connectivity, color-coded results.

These devices offer real-time data and improved convenience, but managing diabetes still requires mastering the basics. Whether you're relying on advanced technology or going back to manual methods during an outage, staying prepared with backup plans, proper supplies, and community support is key to effective diabetes management.

RESOURCES

I've created a dedicated resource page on my website to ensure all tools and templates remain up-to-date and relevant as things change. These resources are based on my personal experiences and are intended to offer guidance and support to families navigating Type 1 diabetes. While every journey is unique, you may find some of the following helpful, along with additional tools and insights:

- Recipe Ideas: Our go-to clean dinner recipes for easy, healthy meals.
- Facebook Group Links: Connect with supportive online communities.
- Community Organizations: Stay engaged with groups like Break Through Type 1.
- Diabetes Supply List: Keep track of essential supplies and expiration dates.
- First Endocrinology Visit Questions: A checklist of key questions to ask.
- Sibling Conversations Guide: Tips for discussing Type 1 diabetes with siblings.
- Classroom Tote Checklist: Must-have items for school classroom kits.
- Emergency Insulin Bag Essentials: A list of what's in my go-to kit.
- Super Sitter Guide: A resource for babysitters caring for a child with Type 1.

- School Prep Guide: Key questions to bring to school meetings.
- Overnight & Travel Guide: Tips and checklists for extended trips.

Please note that the information provided is based on my personal experiences as a parent navigating Type 1 diabetes. It is not intended as medical advice, and I encourage you to consult with your healthcare team for any medical or treatment-related decisions. My hope is that these resources offer practical support, reassurance, and confidence as you navigate your own journey.

REVIEW INQUIRY

Hi, it's Elizabeth here!

I hope you've been enjoying *A Love Greater than Diabetes*, finding it both useful and inspiring. I have a small favor to ask:

Would you consider giving the book a rating or review on the website where you purchased it? Online bookstores are more likely to promote books that have strong reader feedback, and your review could help others discover it.

Here's how you can help:

1. Visit the website where you bought the book.
2. Search for *A Love Greater than Diabetes* or my name.
3. Leave your review—bonus points if you include a picture of yourself holding the book! Photos often increase the chances of your review being highlighted.

Here's something exciting: **with every book purchased, a copy will be donated to a newly diagnosed family to help them navigate their journey with type 1 diabetes.** Your support not only helps spread the word about the book but also directly impacts another family in need.

Thank you for your time and for being part of this mission!

Many thanks in advance,
Elizabeth Kill

WOULD YOU LIKE ELIZABETH KILL TO SPEAK TO YOUR ORGAIZATION?

Book Elizabeth Now!

Elizabeth Kill accepts a limited number of speaking/coaching/training engagements each year. To learn how you can bring her message to your organization, visit greaterthant1d.com.

ACKNOWLEDGMENTS

First and foremost, I want to thank my amazing friend and family physician, Dr. Laurie Marbas. Laurie, you have been with us through every step of this incredible journey, supporting us in more ways than I can even begin to express. You mean the world to our entire family. I still remember when you encouraged me to write this book; at first, I thought you were a little crazy, but now I am endlessly grateful for your nudge to share our story.

To my incredible book coach, Cathy Fyock—thank you for guiding me from ground zero. Your insight, wisdom, and encouragement helped me shape this book into what it is today. I'm so grateful for the time and effort you poured into helping me bring this project to life.

My family—my biggest cheerleaders, always there with love and support. Thank you for stepping in whenever needed and encouraging me to pursue something impactful. You've filled my heart with joy and made this journey meaningful.

To my dedicated editors, Erik Edwards, Kathy Miller Perkins, and Brigette Rhyne—thank you for your attention to detail and thoughtful feedback. And to my wonderful contributors, Kylie Buckner, Shana Rakowsky, Ashley Thompson, and Lindsay Cook, thank you for sharing your knowledge and passion; you added invaluable depth and insight to this book.

A huge thank you to my marketing team at Book Thinkers for encouraging me to step out of my comfort zone and share my journey with so many. And to my publishing team at Ignite Press, thank you for patiently guiding me through the publishing process with kindness and expertise.

Lastly, to my dear friend Jennifer Berluti—thank you for being there every step of the way. You helped me brainstorm, kept my spirits high, and encouraged me to keep going when I needed it most.

I am beyond grateful to all of you. Your unwavering support, insight, and encouragement have brought such joy to this process and pushed me further than I could have gone alone. Thank you for making this dream a reality!

ABOUT THE AUTHOR

Elizabeth Kill is a dedicated author, advocate for type 1 diabetes, and former president of Auld Technologies, LLC. Her leadership in the consumer product labeling industry was marked by hands-on involvement and strong client relationships. Elizabeth is an alumna of the University of Kentucky with a bachelor's in elementary education. She believes that life's challenges offer profound lessons—a perspective deepened when her child was diagnosed with type 1 diabetes. Currently, 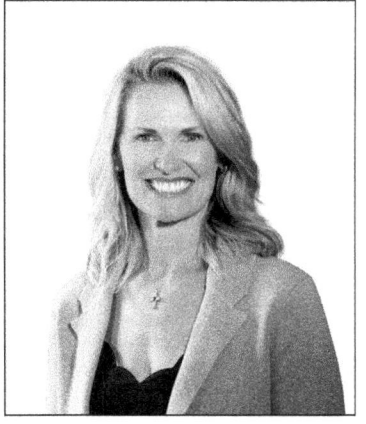 she channels her passion into writing and advocacy, focusing on making a meaningful impact within the type 1 diabetes community. Her work inspires and empowers others, reflecting her commitment to helping those affected by this diagnosis. Elizabeth now resides in Columbus, Ohio, with her husband, Todd, and their children, Marlee Kate and Jackson, where they enjoy adventures together.

Elizabeth can be reached at: elizabeth@greaterthant1d.com.

www.ingramcontent.com/pod-product-compliance
Lightning Source LLC
Chambersburg PA
CBHW070631030426
42337CB00020B/3978